THE DALY DISH RIDES AGAIN

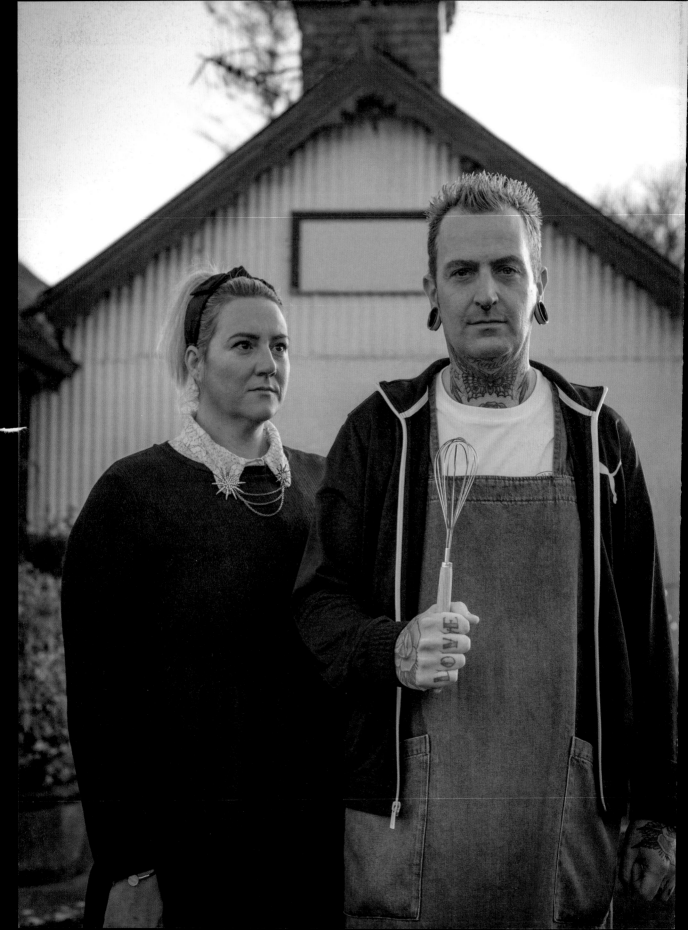

THE DALY DISH RIDES AGAIN

★★★

100
More Masso Slimming Meals for Every Day

★★★

GINA DALY AND MR DISH

GILL BOOKS

Gill Books

Hume Avenue

Park West

Dublin 12

www.gillbooks.ie

Gill Books is an imprint of M.H. Gill and Co.

© Gina Daly 2021

978 07171 9045 4

Designed by www.grahamthew.com

Photography by Leo Byrne

Food styling by Charlotte O'Connell, assisted by Claire Wilkinson

Edited by Susan McKeever

Proofread by Jane Rogers

Indexed by Eileen O'Neill

Printed by Printer Trento S.r.l., Italy

This book is typeset in 10pt Sentinel Light.

The paper used in this book comes from the wood pulp of managed forests.

For every tree felled, at least one tree is planted, thereby renewing natural resources.

A CIP catalogue record for this book is available from the British Library.

5 4 3 2 1

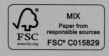

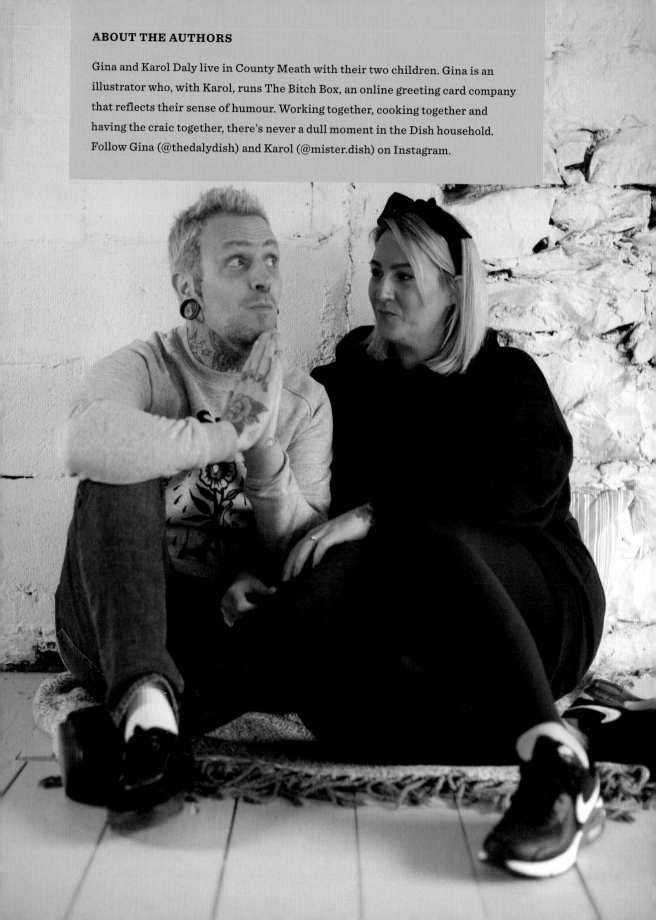

ABOUT THE AUTHORS

Gina and Karol Daly live in County Meath with their two children. Gina is an illustrator who, with Karol, runs The Bitch Box, an online greeting card company that reflects their sense of humour. Working together, cooking together and having the craic together, there's never a dull moment in the Dish household. Follow Gina (@thedalydish) and Karol (@mister.dish) on Instagram.

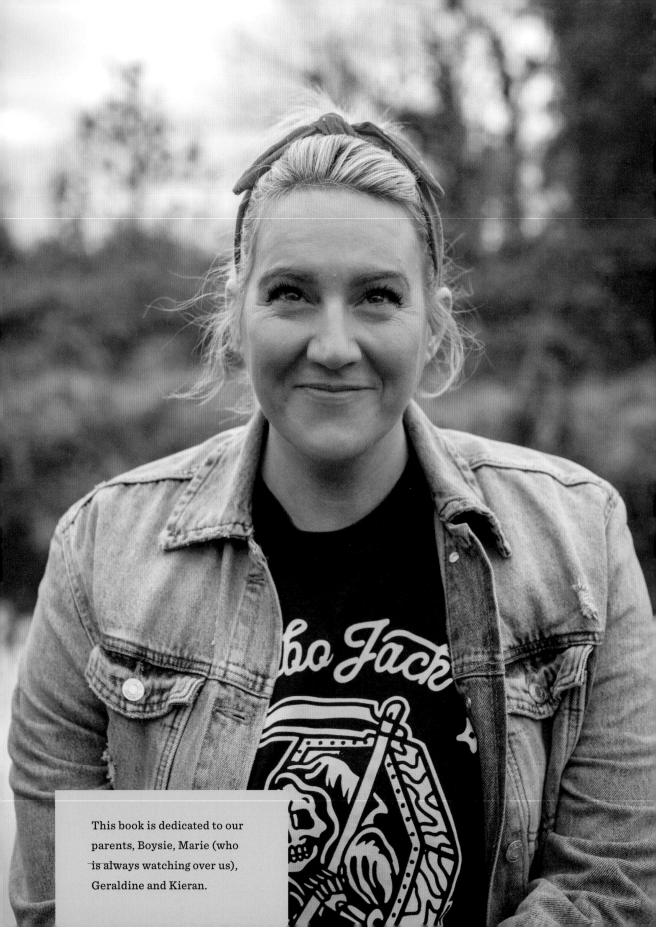

This book is dedicated to our parents, Boysie, Marie (who is always watching over us), Geraldine and Kieran.

✳

CONTENTS

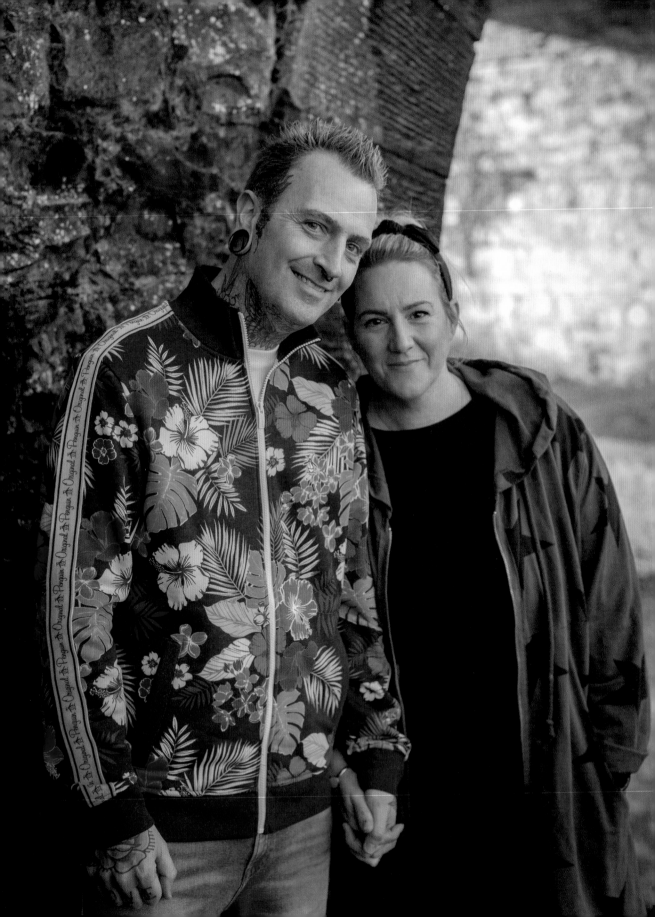

INTRODUCTION

We're back again and we are feckin' delighted!

We are super proud to present to you another deadly cookbook packed to the brim with quick and easy dishes that will have you nearly licking the pages! From breakfast feasts to dinnertime treats, you will find everything you've been looking for between the covers of this book – bigger, bolder and more delicious than before.

Once again, we take our love of audacious, tasty food and keep it on the healthier side with simple store-cupboard ingredients and easy-to-follow steps that the whole family will love and enjoy. As always, our love of the airfryer shines through; but don't worry, it's not essential to make any of these meals – an oven will do the trick – but, in fairness, what have you been doing all your life without one? Lol!

Well, 2020, what a feckin' year. But little did we know the journey we would embark upon, and the fun and exciting things that would happen for us. What started as a little Instagram food diary and a couple cooking at home in their kitchen, just having the craic, has turned into so much more since the release of *The Daly Dish*.

We won't lie, we had the actual fear waiting for our first book to launch. We weren't really known outside our Instagram bubble and we didn't know what way it would go. We had kept the whole project under wraps for months while we were writing and recipe-testing, so when we got the first copy in our hands we were fit to burst with excitement: it was an actual real-life cookbook, with pages 'n' all, and it looked bleedin' deadly!

Then we had the fear of wondering if it would sell. By Jaysus, we could never have imagined what would happen next. Our little book went on to make Irish history, with the highest volume of presales ever recorded, leaving the publishers in a sweat 'cause they quickly sold out of every copy. It went on to be nominated for an An Post Irish Book Award and then, to top it all off, we were the number one bestselling cookbook in Ireland for 2020 – mind-blowing, and all during a pandemic!

Throughout the year, like everyone, we had some great highs and, unfortunately, some painful lows, which left us with heavy hearts. It really brought to light the importance of family and keeping spirits high in a time when we couldn't have our loved ones to hug and hold us and tell us everything would be okay. What did we do to get through it? Well, we cooked, we ate and we shared those family moments around the table that are so important. Even though it was tough, our love of cooking brought us closer, and we have wonderful memories that will last a lifetime.

All the dishes we cooked and shared as a family have now become what you have in your hands: our new book packed full of recipes that come from the heart and a genuine love of good food. We have gotten a little bit more adventurous with these recipes, coming up with some outrageous new dishes that we know you guys will love, but keeping those essential comfort staples in there too.

Now, while we did cook up a storm, and I found myself breezing through lockdown without the 'COVID stone' gain, I then hit a wall and it floored me! My style of cooking had become my lifestyle for so long and it was second nature to me to keep a good balance of healthy eating while still enjoying eating out from time to time, but I lost my momentum after some heart-breaking news. My dad's life partner passed away and I was absolutely devastated for him, and shortly after her passing I found out I had a missed miscarriage. With the restrictions in place my dad never got to say goodbye to his love before she passed away in hospital, and when I was given the news of the miscarriage, I was alone, afraid and felt so empty. It all became too much.

Trying to keep a happy persona on Instagram was tough because behind the camera my heart was broken, for all of us. Grief for me is a funny ole thing. I didn't cry into a tub of Ben & Jerry's; instead, I fed people. I needed to feel the happiness of us all being together, of the chats and the laughs. I needed to forget about the sadness for just a moment and feel the joy of a family meal, whether it was sitting in the car park eating a McDonald's and giggling with the kids while the rain crashed down on the car, or doing the big shop and saying, 'Ah feck it, we'll grab a takeaway on the way home'. Listen, I'm only human – some days it was needed! We don't always need to have our shit together and that's okay. It's okay to 'do you' when you need to and it's also okay to admit that you're not okay.

Needless to say, after I'd taken the time that I needed to recover and ended up with a few new giblets on me legs and thighs (not that I give a shite), I had to take a bit of my own advice. I knew from experience that I lose weight fast but I gain faster, so I quickly jumped back into my old lifestyle of good, hearty, healthy food. As much as my 'time off' to grieve was needed, and it was great to get it out of my system, that feeling of being uncomfortable can bring you down – it's a feckin' catch-22. The important thing is to always remember that a shit week doesn't have to be a shit month, and a shit month doesn't have to be a shit year.

Anyway, time to get cooking! We really hope you guys love this book and the recipes as much as we loved creating them. Enjoy, and happy cooking.

Gina & Karol x

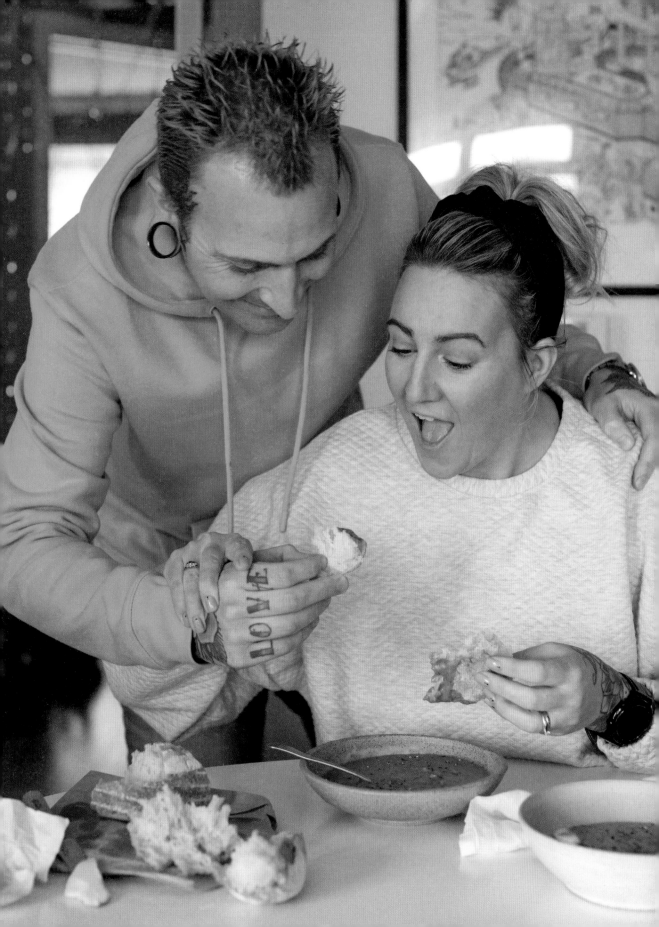

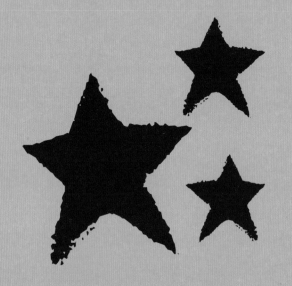

LET'S
GET
LOADED

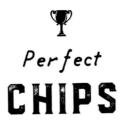

Perfect CHIPS

This is not déjà vu. If you have our first book, this recipe is in there too, I'm just putting it in here for the people in the back who bought them in the wrong order! It's a handy reference and will save you from jumping from book to book as it's a staple recipe. This simple and easy method will give you perfectly crispy and tasty chips every time. I get asked all the time, 'How do you make your chips look so nice?' and honestly, it's so easy that if I can do it, you can too!

SERVES 4

1kg potatoes
Low-calorie spray oil

1 Wash and peel your spuds and cut into chips. I like mine chunky but you can chop them into wedges or French fries.
2 Pop them in a plastic microwave-safe bowl and give them a good rinse under the tap, then you need to drain ALL the water off; this is very important.
3 Pop them in the microwave and cook on full power for 12–13 minutes (less if making a smaller batch), giving them a good shake halfway through. You want them to be soft to the touch, but not mushy. Don't worry if they stick – this is just the starch; you can rinse again in cold water after they are ready and this will unstick them.
4 At this point you can season with paprika or garlic granules, but I like mine plain and simple.
5 Next pop them into the airfryer at 200°C. It will take roughly 15–20 minutes to get your chips nice and golden, but pay attention to my special trick:
6 Every five minutes I open the basket and give the chips a little spray with my oil and a good shake. This ensures they all cook evenly and end up super crispy from the oil. If I'm cooking for a gang and I have to make a few batches, I leave the made ones in a bowl and just as my last batch is ready I throw them all back in together to heat them up. (Just make sure you don't keep eating them while you are waiting, 'cause, trust me, they are feckin' delicious!)

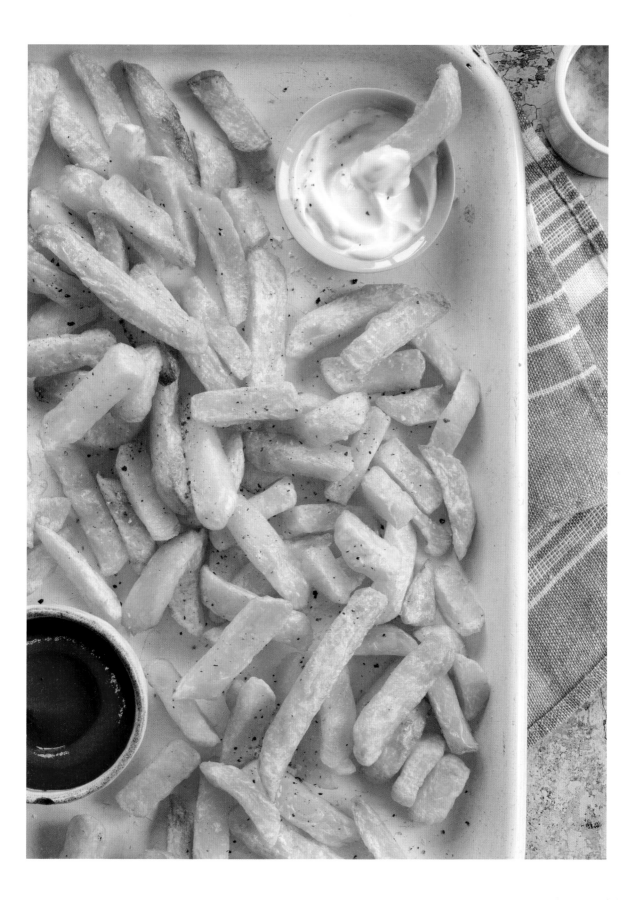

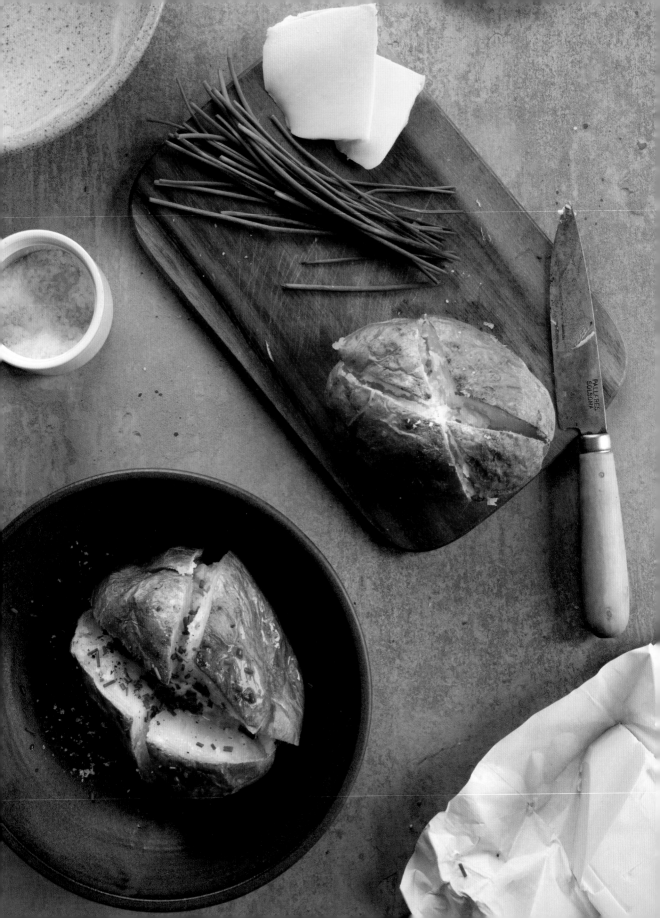

♥

Airfryer
BAKED POTATOES

Loaded high or just with a knob of melting butter, you really cannot go wrong with a baked potato and these are perfect every time! Gorgeous crispy skins and light and fluffy on the inside. Like my chips, I like to make sure that they cook evenly so first I give them a zap in the microwave just to help them along and guarantee they are not like bullets on the inside.

SERVES 4

4 large spuds
Low-calorie spray oil
Sea salt

To serve:

Salty Irish butter
Fresh chives, chopped
Sea salt
Freshly ground black pepper

1 Give your spuds a good scrub – you want the skins to be clean so you can eat them too (it's the best bit). Cut an X into the top of each spud or prick it with a fork.

2 Pop on a microwave-safe plate and put in the microwave for 10 minutes, until slightly tender to touch.

3 Now put them in the airfryer with a little spray of oil and a grind of salt. Cook at 190°C for 25–30 minutes or until golden and crisp and soft to the touch. The size of your airfryer will determine how many spuds you can cook at once, so make sure you don't pile them on top of each other – only add what fits.

4 Once ready, slice the spuds open and add your toppings. For me, nothing beats a bit of butter and some chopped chives; classic and simple. A sprinkle of sea salt and a few grinds of black pepper and you're all set.

Bacon and
CHEESE FRIES

Hands up if you love chips, hands up if you love cheese and bacon ... lash the three together and you will be in heaven.

SERVES 1

2 smoked bacon medallions

250g potatoes

5–6 sprays of low-calorie spray oil

3 light cheese singles, torn

50–100ml water

1 If you are not using an airfryer, preheat the oven to 220°C.

2 Pop the bacon under the grill until golden and crispy, then finely chop and set aside. Wash and peel your spuds and cut into chips, pop in a microwave-safe bowl, then rinse and drain all the water off. Pop in the microwave for 6–7 minutes until slightly soft.

3 Spray the chips with oil and, if using an oven, pop on a baking tray and into the preheated oven for 15–20 minutes. Otherwise put them in the airfryer at 200°C for 15 minutes, shaking and respraying halfway through.

4 To make the cheese sauce, put the cheese singles in a little pot with the water and allow to melt over a medium heat, stirring all the time until smooth.

5 When the chips are ready, tip them into a bowl, drizzle with the masso cheese sauce and sprinkle the crispy bacon on top.

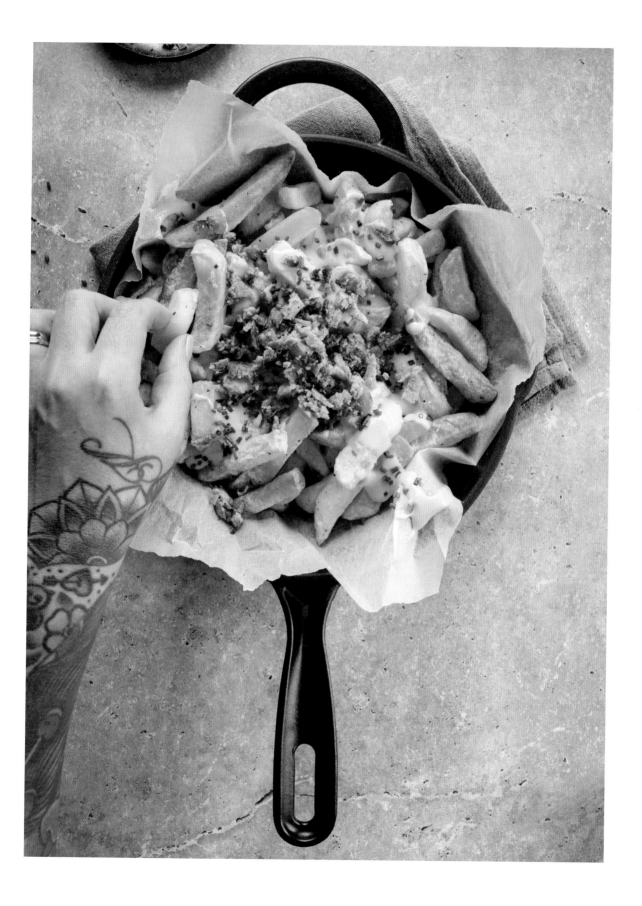

Taco

FRIES

You'll never have to feel like you are missing out ever again with this takeaway essential you can make right in the comfort of your own gaff! Oozy, cheesy goodness with crumbly bacon bits.

SERVES 4

1kg potatoes
Low-calorie spray oil
1 onion, finely diced
500g lean mince
2 tbsp soy sauce
1 tsp easy/lazy garlic
½ tsp easy/lazy chilli
400ml passata
1 tbsp tomato purée
3-4 drops Worcestershire sauce

For the taco sauce:

6 tbsp lighter than light mayo
½ tsp chipotle chilli powder
1 tsp lime juice
½ tsp smoked paprika
½ tsp chilli powder
Water to loosen, if needed

To serve:

Cheddar cheese, grated
A few scallions, thinly sliced

1 If you are not using an airfryer, preheat the oven to 220°C. Wash and peel your spuds and cut into chips, tip into a microwave-safe bowl and rinse and drain thoroughly. Pop into the microwave for 6–7 minutes until slightly soft. Spray the chips with oil, pop on a tray and put in the preheated oven for 15–20 minutes, shaking and turning after 10 minutes, or pop in the airfryer at 200°C for 15 minutes, shaking and respraying halfway through until golden and crisp.

2 While the chips are cooking, heat a little oil in a wok, fry off the onion then add the mince and soy sauce and cook, stirring, until the meat turns brown. Then stir in the garlic and chilli and cook for another 1–2 minutes.

3 Add in the passata, tomato purée and Worcestershire sauce and simmer on a medium heat for 10 minutes until the mixture is starting to reduce.

4 Time to get saucy: mix all the ingredients for the taco sauce together in a bowl.

5 To assemble your taco fries, pop your chips in a bowl and spoon on a layer of the taco mince, drizzle with the taco sauce then sprinkle over some grated Cheddar and scallions ... then mill them!

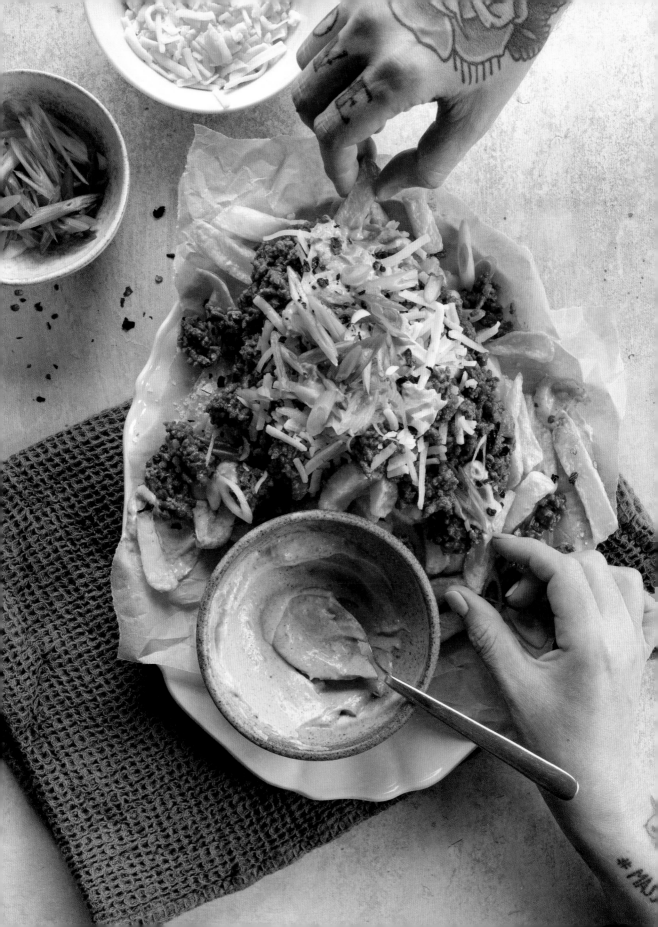

Poutine
FRIES

Here's a little gem of a dish. You can't beat some loaded fries and there are none better than Canadian poutine fries – simply put, these are French fries (chips) loaded up with cheese (traditionally cheese curds) and gravy. As always, we've put our own spin on this Canadian classic. Comforting, tasty and great on their own or as a side dish.

SERVES 2

For the chips:

500g potatoes

Low-calorie spray oil

1 tsp cayenne pepper

1 tsp paprika

For the topping:

150g light mozzarella cheese

200ml Southern Style Gravy (available in supermarkets)

3 scallions, finely chopped

4 slices of ham, cut into small squares

1 If you are not using an airfryer, preheat the oven to 180°C. Wash and peel your spuds and chop into decent-sized chips. Tip into a microwave-safe bowl and rinse and drain thoroughly. Pop into the microwave for around 10–12 minutes, stopping halfway through to give them a good shake. You want them to be soft (not mushy) so they will cook through.

2 Once finished in the microwave, give your chips a couple of sprays with the oil, sprinkle over the cayenne pepper and paprika and give a shake in the bowl to mix everything together.

3 Pop the chips into the airfryer at 200°C for 15–20 minutes. Every 5 or so minutes open the airfryer basket, give a quick spray of oil and give them a shake. You can also pop them on a baking tray and into the preheated oven for the same amount of time, making sure you shake every 5 or so minutes too and spray with the oil.

4 While your chips are cooking, prepare the topping. Get your mozzarella ball, drain off the excess water and slice into thin to medium slices. Make up 200ml of gravy following the instructions on the packet.

5 Get your chips into a bowl and sprinkle over the scallions and ham, then arrange the mozzarella slices evenly around the top.

6 Pop under the grill for a couple of minutes, allowing the cheese to melt in, then pour over the hot gravy and serve.

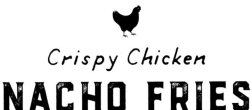

Crispy Chicken

NACHO FRIES

This is a deadly midweek or weekend feast that can be served up in one big dish in the middle of the table for everyone to dig into. Double up the recipe if you have a hungry household – you don't want to run out!

SERVES 2-3

1kg potatoes for chips
Low-calorie spray oil
30g panko breadcrumbs
1 tbsp lemon pepper
2–3 chicken breasts, cut into strips

For the nacho cheese sauce:

3 light cheese singles, torn
1 tbsp hot sauce
50–100 ml water

To serve:

Iceberg lettuce, shredded
1 salad tomato, diced
1 white onion, finely diced
Sliced jalapeños, from a jar

1 If not using an airfryer, preheat the oven to 200°C.

2 First sort your fries out. Follow the instructions for Perfect Chips on page 6.

3 Mix the panko and lemon pepper in a bowl. Spray your chicken strips with a little oil and dip into the seasoned crumbs to coat evenly. You can now either pop them on a baking tray sprayed with a little oil and into the preheated oven for 20 minutes, or, you guessed it, pop into the airfryer at 190°C for 12 minutes or until golden and crispy.

4 Meanwhile, make up the nacho cheese sauce. Pop the cheese singles, hot sauce and water in a little pot on a medium heat and keep stirring until the sauce is smooth and blended.

5 Now, when the chips and chicken are ready to rock, lay a bed of shredded lettuce on a serving dish, load up your crispy chicken and fries then sprinkle the tomato, onion and jalapeños over the top. Finish by drizzling with the sexy cheesy nacho sauce. OMG, divine!

Garlic
PARMESAN FRIES

Here's another quick and tasty recipe for loaded fries – this time just lightly loaded. Simple and tasty, another fave in our house.

SERVES 2

500g potatoes
Low-calorie spray oil
1 tsp garlic granules
60g Parmesan cheese, grated
1 tbsp fresh parsley, chopped
Salt and pepper to taste

1 If you are not using an airfryer, preheat the oven to 180°C. Wash and peel your spuds and chop into nice skinny chips. Get them into a microwave-safe bowl and rinse and drain thoroughly. Pop into the microwave for around 10–12 minutes, stopping halfway through to give them a good shake. You want them to be soft (not mushy) so they will cook through.

2 Give the chips a couple of sprays with the oil, sprinkle over the garlic granules, pop on a tray and put in the preheated oven for 15–20 minutes. You can also pop them in the airfryer at 200°C for 15 minutes, shaking and respraying every 5 minutes.

3 When the chips are cooked, divide them between two bowls, then top with the Parmesan, a sprinkle of parsley and some salt and pepper.

Bacon, Cheese and
SCALLION MASH

This is an exciting, fun take on classic mashed potatoes. We had something similar in a restaurant and it was absolutely gorgeous so I decided to do my own version of it. It's deadly served with a steak or some sausages and gravy. Real comfort food.

SERVES 2

500g potatoes

1 garlic clove, peeled

4 bacon medallions, roughly chopped

1 tsp rapeseed oil

40g red Cheddar cheese, grated

2 scallions, sliced and separated into small circles

Salt and pepper to taste

70ml low-fat milk

1 Peel your potatoes, chop them in half, pop into a pot of salted, boiling water and simmer over a medium heat for around 15–20 minutes. You want them to be nice and soft for mashing.

2 While the potatoes are on the boil, get your garlic and slice into thin slices, and cut your bacon into small squares. Put a pan on a medium heat and add your oil, then add in your garlic. Give it a minute or so just to infuse with the oil and then add in the bacon and fully cook. Once the bacon is cooked put it to one side.

3 Once your spuds are ready to mash, drain off the water and give them a good mash until smooth. Add in the cheese, scallions and salt and pepper, place on a low heat and gradually add in your milk, mixing everything together as you go. You want a nice creamy texture but you don't want it too watery. Once you've a good consistency add in the bacon and give another minute or so on the heat, mixing everything together.

4 You're then good to go. Serve and enjoy.

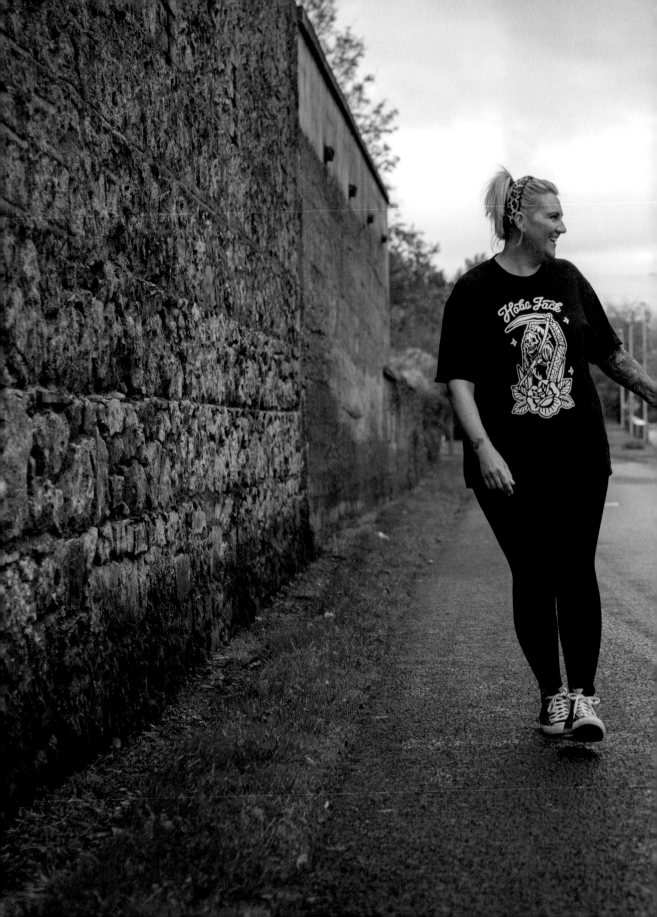

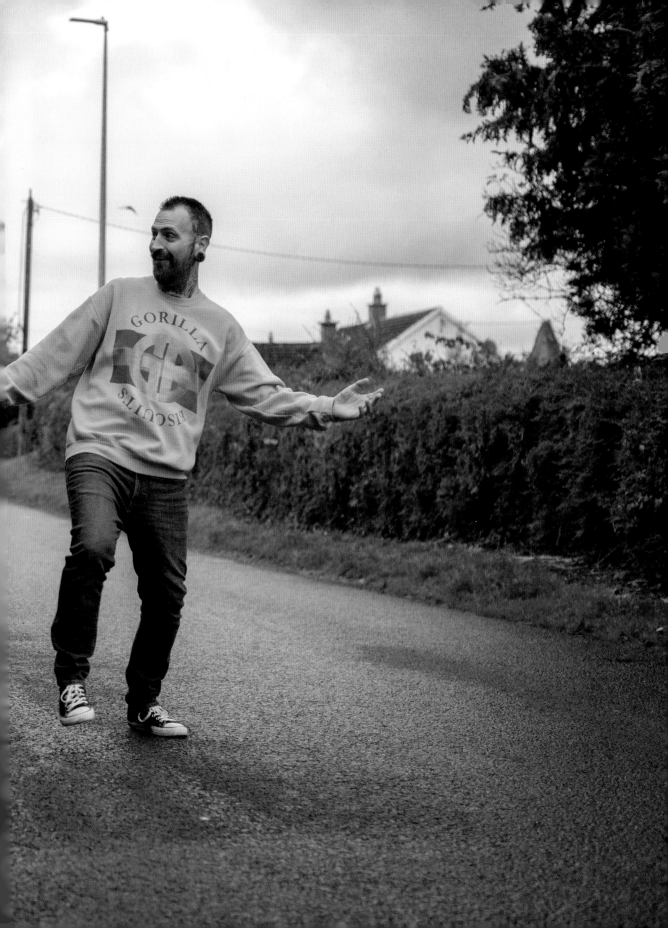

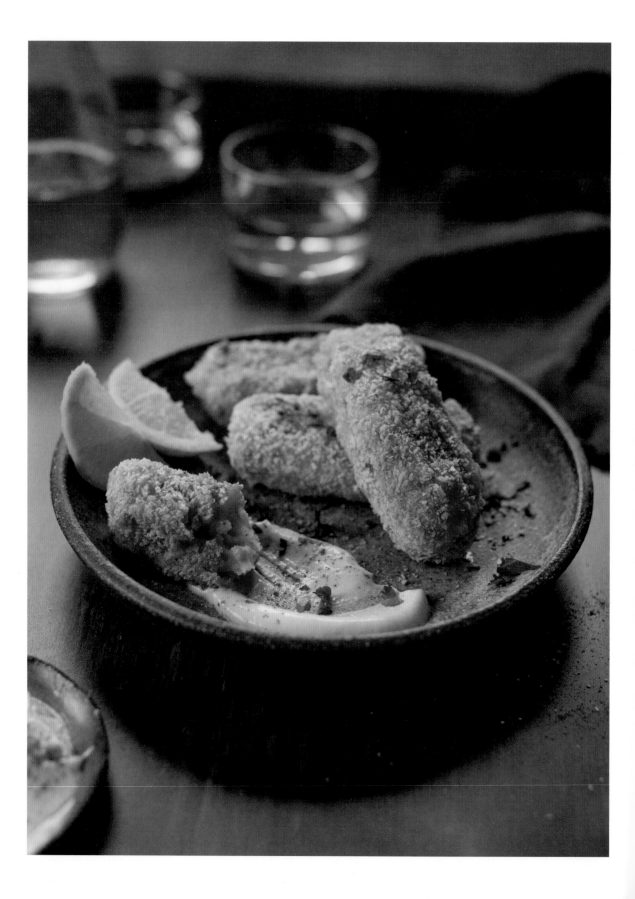

Bacon, Onion and Cheddar
CROQUETTES

If you are like me and make enough mashed potato to feed the neighbourhood, this is a super little way to use up any of that extra that you might have. You can add anything you like to these but I like to use bacon, onion and cheese in mine. You can prepare them in advance and heat them when needed. And best of all, the kids love them too!

SERVES 4

4 smoked bacon medallions
Low-calorie spray oil
½ a small onion, finely diced
250g leftover mash
30g Cheddar cheese, grated
Salt to taste

For the coating:

40g instant mash or panko breadcrumbs
1 tsp turmeric
¼ tsp white pepper
Salt to taste
Low-calorie spray oil

1 If you are not using an airfryer, preheat the oven to 200°C. Grill the bacon until golden and crisp, then chop it up super-fine.

2 Fry off the onion in a pan with a spray of oil until translucent and add this to the cold mashed potato, along with the bacon bits, Cheddar cheese and some salt to taste.

3 Spray some greaseproof paper with low-calorie spray and spoon out about 3 tablespoons of the mixture per croquette. Shape in to cylinder shapes or balls – whatever floats your boat – and leave aside while you get on with the coating.

4 In a bowl, mix the instant mash or panko with the turmeric, white pepper and salt to taste – the turmeric will give your croquettes a nice yellow colour.

5 Spray the croquettes with a little oil then roll in the coating until fully covered. Once coated, spray with some more oil, pop on a baking tray and cook in the preheated oven for 20 minutes, turning halfway through. If you have an airfryer you can pop them in there for 15 minutes at 200°C until golden and crisp.

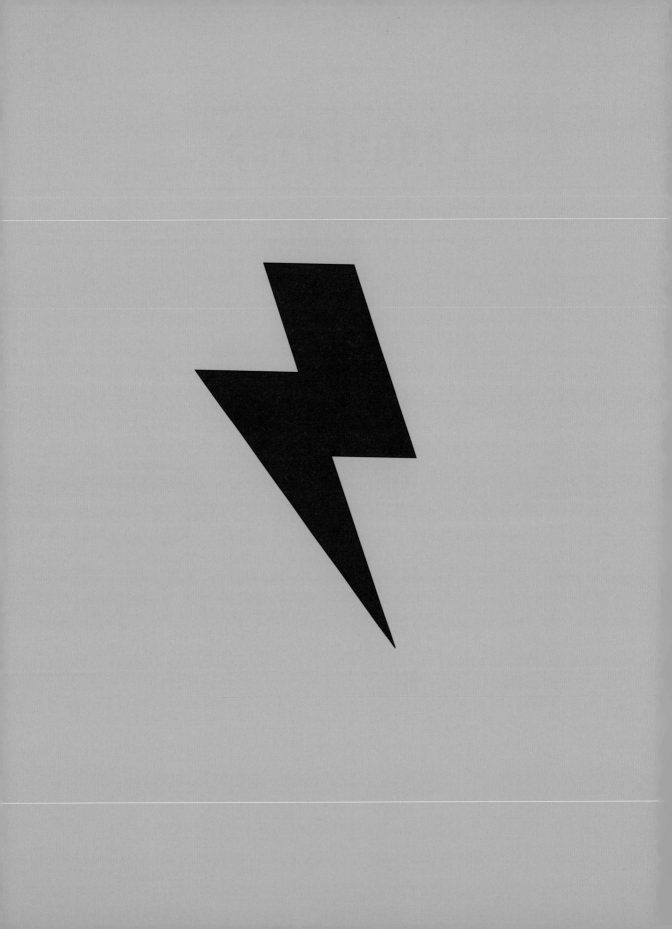

CURRY
IN A
HURRY

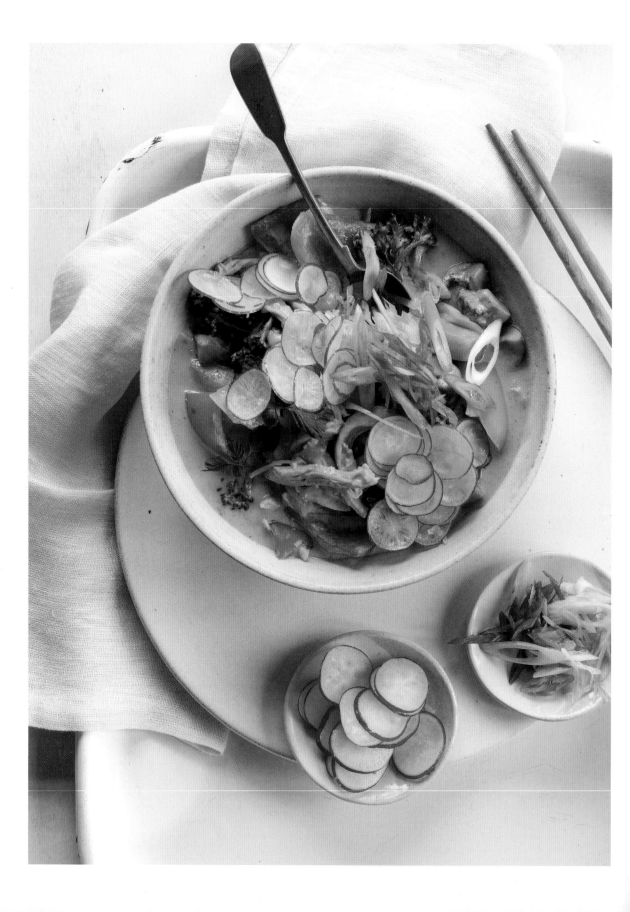

Coconut

CURRY

We LOVE this curry! It's fresh, it's fragrant, it's creamy and, best of all, it's packed full of veggies. We like to up the veggie intake even more by serving it with cauliflower rice (see page 174).

SERVES 4

Low-calorie spray oil

1 onion, finely chopped

4 garlic cloves, minced

2 carrots, sliced or grated

8–10 mushrooms, quartered

1 red pepper, deseeded and roughly chopped

1 yellow pepper, deseeded and roughly chopped

½ head of fresh broccoli, chopped

400ml reduced-fat coconut milk

300ml slimline milk

1 tsp turmeric

2 tsp medium curry powder

½ chicken stock pot

1 tsp cornflour

3–4 chicken breasts, cooked and shredded (see page 158)

To garnish:

2–3 scallions, finely sliced

4 radishes, thinly sliced

1 In a high-sided pan or wok, heat a little spray oil and fry off the onion and garlic until the onion is translucent. Add in the carrots, mushrooms, peppers and broccoli, and stir for 3–5 minutes.

2 Add in the coconut milk, milk, turmeric and curry powder and stir well, then add your half chicken stock pot directly in. Allow to dissolve in the liquid, stirring to mix.

3 Bring the sauce to a boil, then reduce the heat and simmer for 10 minutes until it starts to thicken. If it doesn't thicken to your liking, mix the cornflour in a cup with 1 tsp water and add it into the sauce to help it along.

4 Add in the cooked shredded chicken, heat it through in the sauce, and your curry is ready! Serve on a bed of cauliflower rice and garnish with the sliced scallions and radishes.

Chicken

ROGAN JOSH WRAP

Back when I was in my twenties I used to work in an office and down the road from us there was this awesome little deli that I frequently visited for lunch. They didn't just do the normal regular lunch stuff, they had a couple of different types of curries that they would serve in a warm wrap, which were just divine. Here's my throwback to one of my old lunchtime faves, although this can be served as a dinner too – even add in a little rice to bulk it up.

SERVES 2

1 tbsp rapeseed oil

1 white onion, finely chopped

2 garlic cloves, crushed

2 chicken fillets, diced

2 tbsp rogan josh curry paste

2 tbsp tomato purée

6 cherry tomatoes, quartered

1 tsp chilli flakes (only if you want it spicy)

3 tbsp Greek yoghurt

½ a butterhead lettuce, washed and leaves separated

2 wholemeal wraps

A small handful of fresh coriander, chopped

1 lime, halved

1 Grab your wok and add in the oil, onion and garlic and cook for a couple of minutes on a medium heat. Then throw in your chicken and cook through, moving it around the pan, until nice and brown.

2 Add in your paste, tomato purée, cherry tomatoes and chilli flakes and continue to cook for a couple of minutes, stirring everything together. Lastly add in your yoghurt and stir through.

3 Heat your wraps in the microwave or oven and line with the lettuce then add the saucy chicken, sprinkle over the coriander, and finish with a squeeze of fresh lime. Wrap up and enjoy. You can also serve this piled on top of some warmed naan, as pictured.

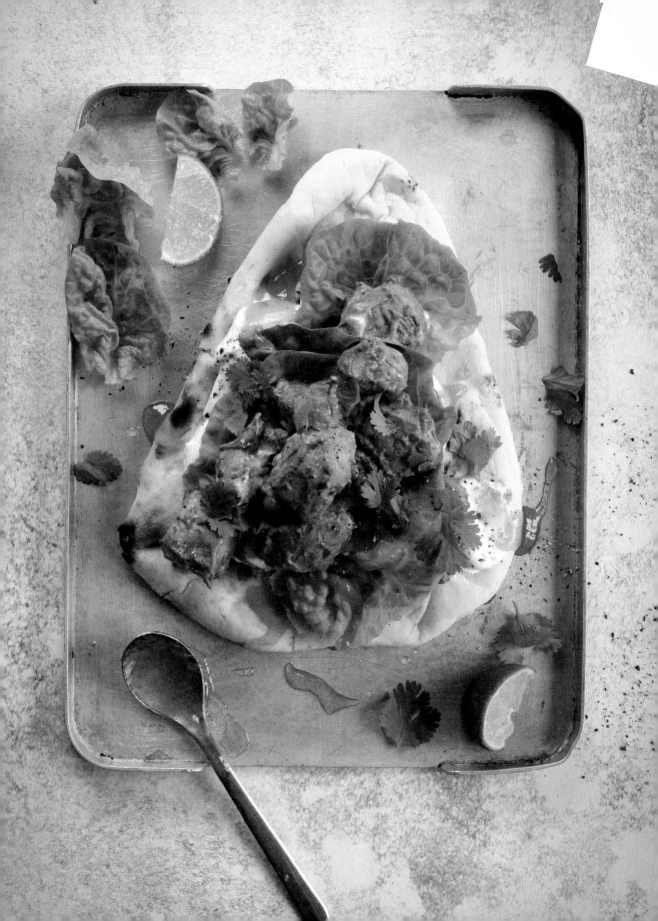

KORMA

This easy chicken korma is perfect for the whole family – mild, creamy and dreamy and perfect for a Friday night fake make. Add some naan bread or poppadoms on the side to dunk and some pilau rice to complete the feast.

SERVES 4

Low-calorie spray oil

1 onion, finely diced

2 garlic cloves, minced

3–4 chicken fillets, diced

2 tbsp korma spice

200ml chicken stock

200ml coconut milk

200ml almond milk

1 tbsp tomato purée

1 tsp sweetener

2 tsp cornflour (optional)

1 Heat a wok or high-sided pan with a little oil, add the onion and garlic and fry off for 2–3 minutes until softened.

2 Add in the diced chicken and brown, stirring to cook every piece evenly. When the chicken is cooked, sprinkle on the korma spice and heat through.

3 Add the chicken stock, coconut milk, almond milk, tomato purée and sweetener. Give it a good stir and bring the sauce to a boil, then reduce the heat and let simmer for 10 minutes. At this stage the sauce should start to reduce and thicken, but if it doesn't thicken as much as you would like, mix the cornflour with some water to a paste and add it into the sauce.

4 We like to serve ours with basmati rice, warmed naan bread and poppadoms to dunk – nothing like it!

Banging

BOMBAY POTATOES

Another awesome little Indian dish, perfect for a side dish, starter or even a flavour-packed snack. These also go great with a curry as an alternative to rice.

SERVES 2

500g potatoes

1 tsp sea salt

1 tsp turmeric

1 tsp garam masala

1 tsp smoked paprika

1 tsp ground cumin

1 tsp garlic granules

1 tbsp oil (I use rapeseed oil)

Salt and pepper to taste

1 If you are not using an airfryer, preheat the oven to 180°C.

2 Wash and peel your potatoes and chop into nice even cubes. Boil them in a pot of boiling water with the salt and turmeric for around 15 minutes, until cooked.

3 Next up, drain your spuds well and put into a mixing bowl. Add in the garam masala, smoked paprika, cumin and garlic granules. Finally drizzle over the oil.

4 Using your (clean) hands, mix everything together, coating the potatoes evenly with everything.

5 Place the spiced potatoes on a baking tray and into the preheated oven, or into an airfryer at 180°C, for 12–15 minutes, checking every 4 minutes or so and giving them a shake.

6 Add a little salt and pepper and serve.

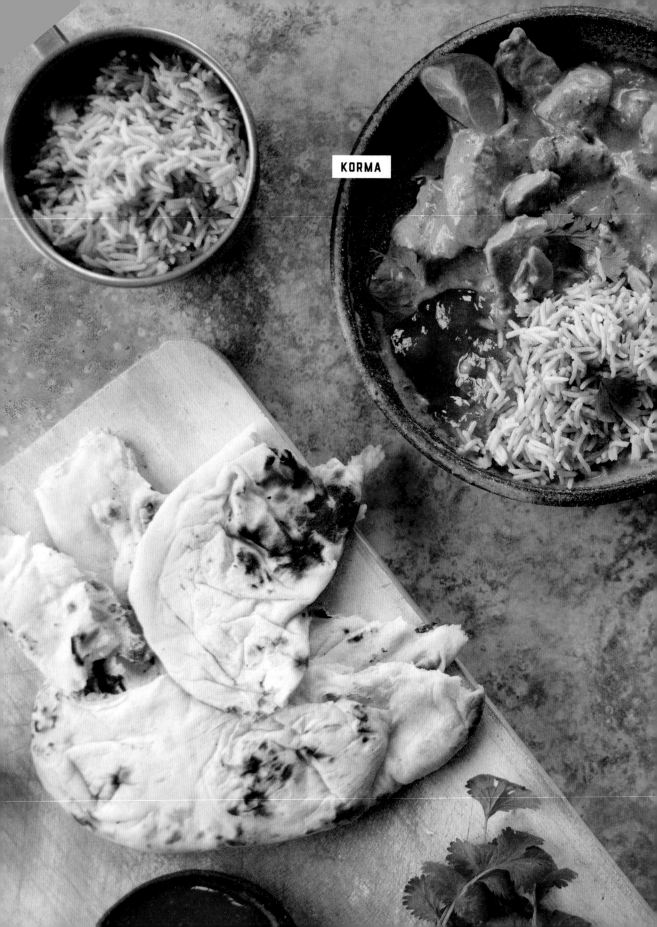

KORMA

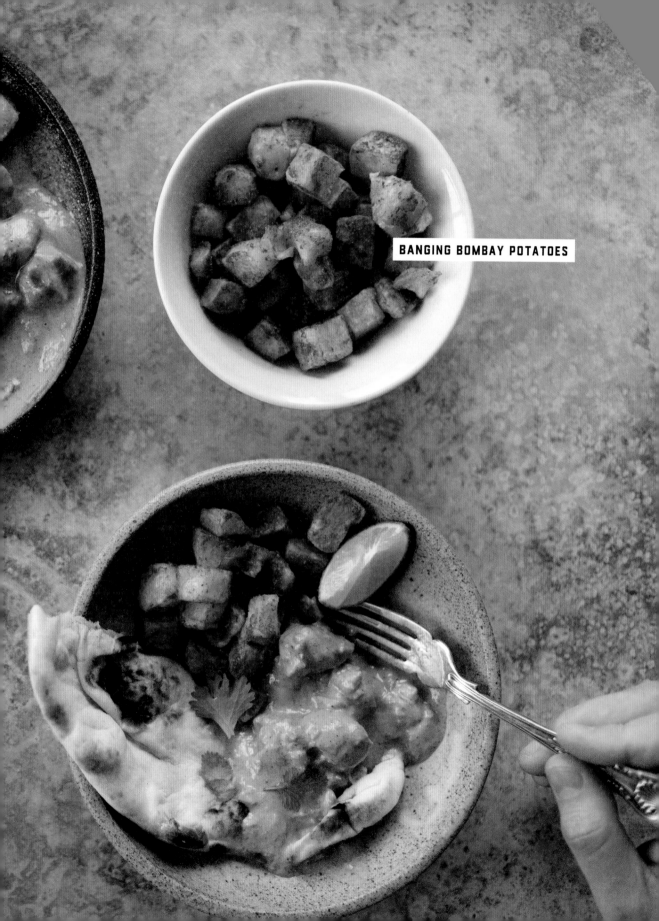

BANGING BOMBAY POTATOES

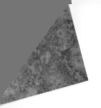

Coconut and
TOMATO CURRY

I don't know about anyone else but we have a few curry nights in our house each week. Everything you need is probably sitting in your cupboard just waiting to be used and your curry will be ready in no time at all. This is a fab little recipe that is sweet and tangy but has a nice little warm kick.

SERVES 4

4 large chicken fillets

Low-calorie spray oil

Veg of your choice: I like onion and green peppers, sliced

For the sauce:

2 tsp yellow curry paste

1 tsp garlic purée

1 x 400g tin of chopped tomatoes

300ml light coconut milk

1 tbsp soy sauce

1 tsp fish sauce

1 tbsp sweet chilli sauce

1 I like to boil the chicken for this recipe. Put the whole fillets in a large pot of boiling water and let them simmer for 15–20 minutes until cooked through. Remove from the water, then use a couple of forks to shred the chicken. Set aside while you prepare your veg of choice.

2 In a wok or high-sided pan, spray a little oil, add in your sliced veg and cook through until just tender. Remove from the pan and pop aside while you prepare your sauce.

3 Heat the curry paste in the wok or high-sided pan for 1–2 minutes, then add the garlic purée and the tin of tomatoes. Stir and heat for 5 minutes, then add in the rest of the ingredients.

4 Bring up the heat to a boil, add in the shredded chicken and cooked vegetables and mix well, then turn down the heat and allow to simmer gently for 10 minutes.

5 Serve on a bed of boiled rice.

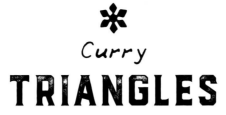

Curry
TRIANGLES

I used to work waiting tables in a Chinese restaurant years and years ago. It was one of those all-you-can-eat buffet-style places and the food was fabulous, and at the end of the night they would dish out the leftover food for us to take home so it didn't go to waste. As much as I loved the main dishes, I was all about the 'nibbly bits' – aka the starters – and would bring home all the curry triangles and spring rolls. I'm still all about the nibbly bits but now I love to make my own healthier versions. This one is a banger and super-easy to recreate!

SERVES 4

Low-calorie spray oil

300g leaner option mince

½ an onion, finely chopped

1 garlic clove, minced

1 tsp mild curry powder

100ml water

2 tbsp frozen petits pois

1 tsp cornflour

Filo pastry sheets

1 Preheat the oven to 200°C.

2 Start with your filling. Spray a little oil on a pan and add the mince, onion and garlic and fry off until the onion is translucent and the mince is browned.

3 Add in the curry powder and water and stir in the peas, mixing for 2–3 minutes until the peas cook through and the liquid reduces. We want to thicken the liquid a little so mix your cornflour to a paste in a cup with a little water and add this in.

4 Cook for another few minutes until your sauce has thickened well (you don't want it spreading all over the pastry) then pop to one side and allow to cool.

5 To prepare the pastry, separate the sheets and cut in half (if you want the pastry thicker you can fold each sheet in half and use it all).

6 I use half a sheet per triangle. Lay out a pastry piece on a board, then put 1 tablespoon of the mince mixture in the top-left corner and fold the pastry diagonally over it to form a triangle. Continue folding over and over to form a triangle that is roughly palm-sized.

7 Repeat with remaining filo sheets and mince mixture.

8 Spray each triangle with oil, pop on a baking tray and into the preheated oven and cook for 12–15 minutes or until golden and crisp. You can also pop them in the airfryer at 190°C for 7–8 minutes.

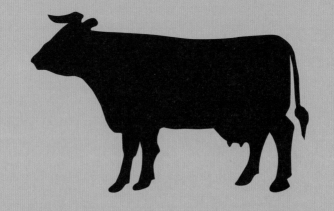

BADASS
BURGERS

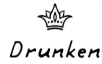

Drunken
CHICKEN BURGER

With a name like 'drunken chicken burger' you know it's going to be a good one! This is great for when you fancy a takeaway but would prefer to make your own healthier version. There's a lot going on with flavour here – the chilli, maple and bourbon all work really well together and give an epic taste sensation. And remember, this is a HOT one. You'll need to have some zombie slaw to hand (see page 73) to assemble these bad boys.

SERVES 2

1 egg

30g Chilli Heatwave Doritos

2 chicken fillets

Low-calorie spray oil

6 fresh jalapeño peppers

For the sauce:

4 tbsp maple syrup (plus some to drizzle on the jalapeños)

2 tbsp bourbon

To build your burgers:

2 wholemeal buns

2 tbsp zombie slaw

½ a head of lettuce, leaves separated

1 First off, crack your egg into a bowl and give it a good whisk. Grab your Doritos and smash up in a pestle and mortar (or put into a plastic bag and bash them up). Once crushed, pop into a separate bowl.

2 Butterfly your fillets: place on a board, slice into one side, but not completely in half. Open up the breast into a 'butterfly' shape. Dip each butterflied fillet first into the egg, then into the crushed Doritos. You want them nice and coated here, so use your hands to press on the Dorito crumbs. Give them a light spray with the oil and pop into an airfryer at 180° for 15 minutes, turning halfway through. Alternatively pop onto a frying pan on a medium heat for 15 minutes, turning halfway through.

3 While your chicken is cooking, grab your jalapeños, chop off the stems and slice lengthways down the middle. Line them all up on a baking tray lined with greaseproof paper, drizzle over a little maple syrup and pop into the preheated oven for around 5–7 minutes – keep an eye on them.

4 To make the sauce, get your maple syrup and bourbon into a pot and put on a low to medium heat, stirring well to mix as it heats up.

5 When your chicken is cooked up grab your buns and lightly toast them, put some zombie slaw on each bottom bun, followed by the roasted jalapeños. Place your chicken fillet on top and, using a spoon, drizzle half the sauce mix over each one, followed by the lettuce and top bun.

6 You might have sticky fingers after eating this but you won't be hungry.

Fillet O' Fish
BURGER

Here's a handy one for a quick and healthy lunch or perfect for a dinner served alongside some homemade chips (see page 6). It's also a great one for the kids and definitely a healthy alternative to a takeout or frozen fish burgers.

SERVES 2

20g golden breadcrumbs
(available in supermarkets)

1 tbsp lemon pepper

Salt and pepper

1 egg

2 cod fillets

Low-calorie spray oil

2 wholemeal burger buns

2 light cheese slices

1 gherkin, sliced

1 Preheat the oven to 180°C.

2 Get your breadcrumbs and lemon pepper into a mixing bowl, add a sprinkle of salt and pepper then mix together. In a separate bowl, crack your egg and whisk it.

3 Dunk your cod fillets first into the egg mix, coating both sides, then into the breadcrumb mix, making sure each fillet is well coated with the crumbs.

4 Give both fillets a spray of oil then place on a baking tray and into the preheated oven for 12–15 minutes, turning halfway through.

5 While these are cooking, get your buns toasted. When the fish fillets are ready, layer them up on the buns with a slice of cheese and some gherkin.

6 Another great addition to this is some of our tarty sauce (recipe on page 141 of our first book, *The Daly Dish*).

Cheeseburger
SPRING ROLLS

When you love an aul cheeseburger but equally love a spring roll this is the perfect marriage of two of your loves. I first had these in a really cool bar in Dublin and my head literally blew off my shoulders when I bit into them! I was curious ordering, I was dubious before taking my first bite, but I was sold as soon as I tasted them! Sweet divine, they were such a taste sensation I knew I would have to create my own version. I'm taking the cheeseburger taco recipe (cause that's just massive), minus one or two bits, and rolling it into crispy bites of heaven. You are going to bleedin' love these, trust me. Ohh and let's have a homemade burger sauce for dipping for good measure – feck it!

SERVES 8

Low-calorie spray oil

½ an onion, finely chopped

500g lean mince

30ml water

1 tsp garlic granules

½ tsp chilli flakes

3–4 drops Worcestershire sauce

1 tbsp tomato purée

2 tbsp soy sauce

3 cherry tomatoes, chopped

1–2 gherkins, chopped

A pinch of salt

3 slices American cheese singles, torn

Filo pastry sheets or 8 spring roll wrappers (available from Asian supermarkets)

Cheddar cheese, grated

Sesame seeds

For the dipping sauce:

1 tbsp tomato ketchup

1 tbsp Caesar sauce

1 tsp American yellow mustard

1 pickled gherkin, finely chopped

1 tsp gherkin juice

1 If not using an airfryer, preheat the oven to 200°C.

2 Grab a wok or high-sided pan, spray with some oil and fry off the onion until it's translucent, then add the mince with the water (this will stop it clumping together). Stir until brown.

3 When the mince is cooked through, add in the garlic granules and chilli flakes, the Worcestershire sauce, tomato purée and soy sauce, mix well, and cook for a further 2–3 minutes.

4 Add in your chopped tomatoes and gherkins and mix through. Then add the salt and the cheese singles, let the cheese melt in and mix to combine everything together.

5 If using filo pastry, cut each sheet in half to make squares. Place a good portion of the mince mix in the centre of your wrapper of choice, and a sprinkle of Cheddar cheese. Make sure you leave a good gap all around the mince.

6 Now imagine the wrapper as a clock so I can tell you how to fold it:

- 12 o'clock is pointing away from you.
- 6 o'clock is pointing towards you.
- 3 o'clock is the right side.
- 9 o'clock is the left side.

Fold the left and right sides towards the centre.

7 Then lift the 6 o'clock flap, bring it over the top of the filling and the tucked bits ... stick it down just behind the filling (kind of tuck it) and start to roll it until it's all nice and tidy, stuck together and looking like a spring roll, and that's it! Repeat this process with the remaining wrappers.

8 As the meat is already cooked through, we are really just looking to crisp up the pastry. First I sprinkle over some sesame seeds to make them pretty, then I pop the rolls in the airfryer with a light spray of oil for 6–7 minutes at 180°C until golden brown (or you can pop them in the preheated oven for 15 minutes).

9 To make the dipping sauce, mix all the ingredients (except the pickle juice) together in a glass. It should be a nice peachy colour. Finish by stirring in the pickle juice.

10 When the spring rolls are ready dip them into the sauce to your heart's content!

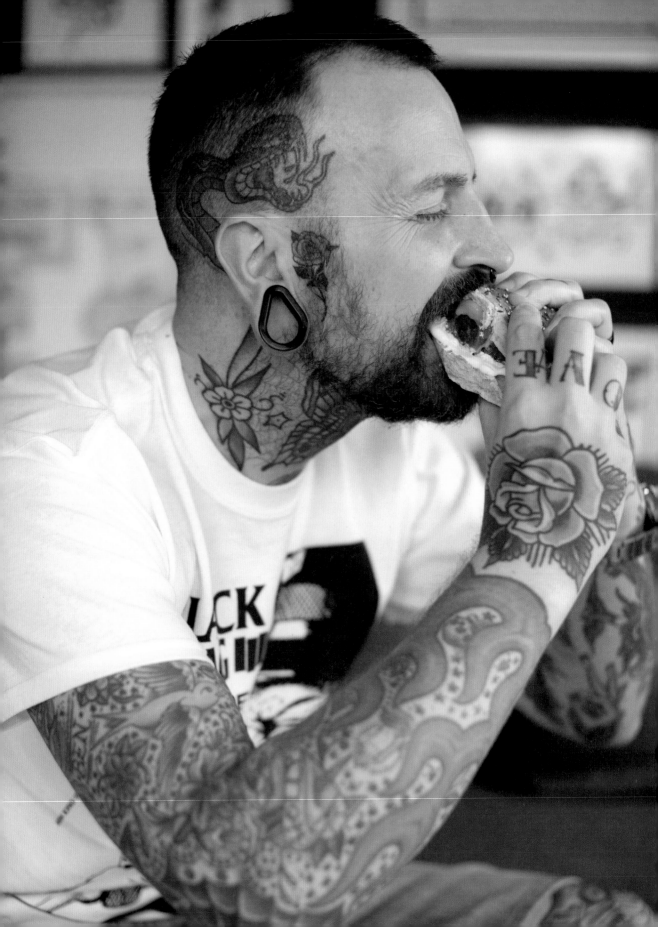

Lamb

BURGER

If you're looking for something a little different, these are definitely worth a try. They're juicy, packed with flavour and are a nice change-up from a regular burger. They were a huge hit with the kids! If you find that the toppings are too much for little mouths, try serving with some cheese and a little ketchup.

SERVES 2

300g lean lamb mince

1 tsp Lebanese 7 spice

1 tsp garlic granules

1 tsp smoked paprika

Salt and pepper to taste

Low-calorie spray oil

30g Cheddar cheese, sliced

30g mozzarella cheese, sliced

To build the burgers:

2 wholemeal buns

2–3 tbsp sour cream

2 large tomatoes, thickly sliced

1 onion, thickly sliced

2–3 tbsp shop-bought salsa verde (optional)

1 Get your lamb mince into a mixing bowl and add in the 7 spice, garlic granules, smoked paprika and a pinch of salt and pepper. Using your (clean) hands, give everything a good mix together, then form two burger patties – use a burger press if you have one, or if not you can use the bottom of a plate to flatten.

2 Give a couple of sprays of oil to a pan, get it on a medium heat and pop the burgers onto it, cooking for around 5–7 minutes on each side.

3 When the burgers are cooked, pop the Cheddar and mozzarella on top of the burgers on the pan and cover with a bowl for around a minute – you want the cheese to get all nice and melted. Another option is to pop them under the grill for a minute.

4 Lightly toast your buns and start by spreading the sour cream on the bottom, followed by the burger patty, then your tomato and onion and lastly your salsa verde, if you have it. Pop the top bun on and enjoy.

Maple

CHICKEN BURGER

At this point you've probably guessed that I am a huge burger fan. I can't get enough and the chicken fillet burger is always a satisfying feed. With this one we're going for a little sweet and sour vibe to give a great balance of flavour, making for one epic burger.

SERVES 2

1 egg

30g panko breadcrumbs

1 tbsp lemon pepper

2 chicken fillets

Low-calorie spray oil

4 bacon medallions

4 tbsp maple syrup

½ tsp ground cinnamon

To build the burgers:

2 wholemeal buns

2 tbsp Frank's RedHot Buffalo Wings Sauce (available in supermarkets)

½ a head of lettuce, leaves separated

2 gherkins, sliced into rounds

1 Get yourself two bowls, crack your egg into one and give it a whisk, then put your breadcrumbs and lemon pepper into the other and mix it up.

2 Grab your fillets and butterfly them (see page 36), then one by one dip them first into the egg and then into the breadcrumbs, making sure to get both sides evenly covered.

3 You can either cook the fillets in the airfryer (15 minutes at 180°C) or on the pan – I usually do them on the pan for about 5–7 minutes each side. For either cooking method give your fillets a couple of sprays of oil before cooking.

4 While the chicken is on, grab your bacon medallions and slice them into small strips lengthways, kinda like mini bacon fries. Pop them on another small pan with a spray of oil and cook on a medium heat for a couple of minutes until fully cooked and crisping up. While the bacon bits are cooking I usually add a teaspoon of maple syrup to the pan and mix up just to give them a light coating.

5 Get your maple syrup into a pot, add in the cinnamon and put on a low heat for a couple of minutes until warmed up, then get ready to build your burger.

6 Toast your buns, then add a tablespoon of the Frank's sauce to each bottom bun and spread out, following up with the lettuce.

7 Next grab your chicken fillets (one at a time) and pour over half the maple and cinnamon sauce – as much of it as possible. I usually do this over the pan as it can be messy.

8 Then add the fillet to the bun and top that with the bacon, sliced gherkin, and finally the top bun.

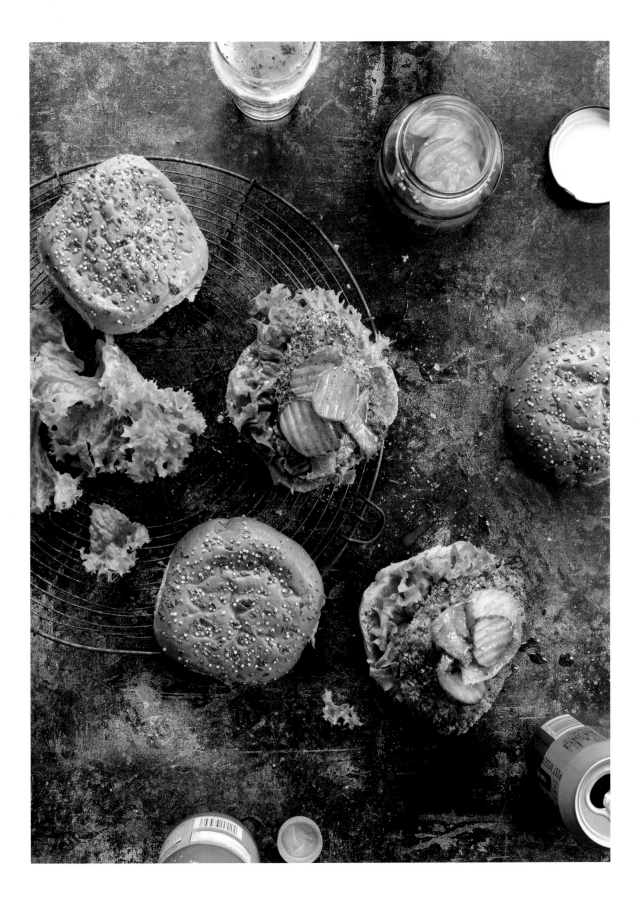

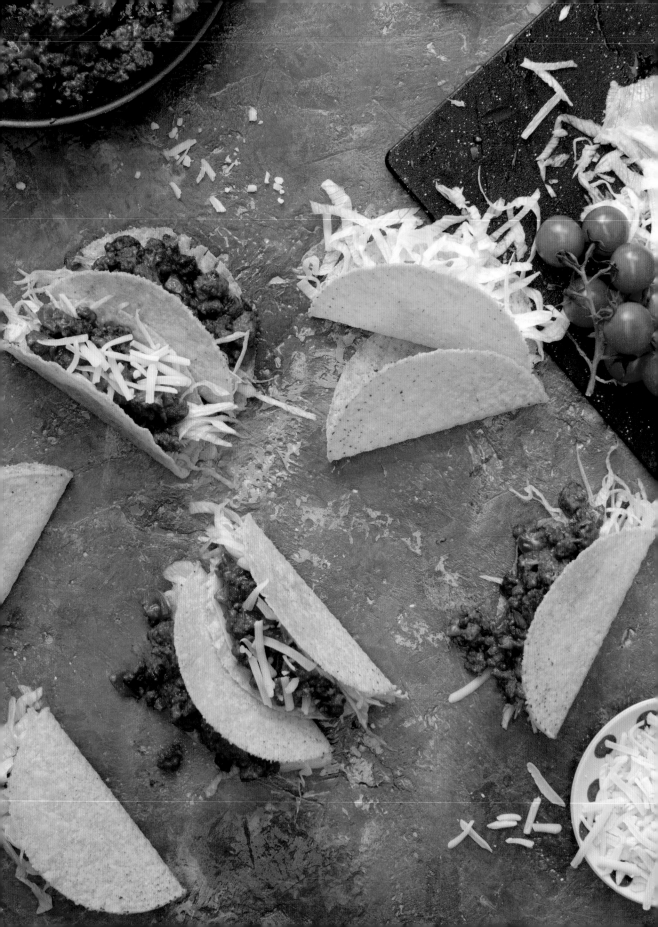

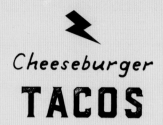

Cheeseburger
TACOS

Just when you thought a cheeseburger couldn't get any ridier, the cheeseburger taco came along and blew your mind. It's everything you ever wanted from a cheeseburger, but loaded into a crispy taco shell for extra crunch.

SERVES 4–6

Low-calorie spray oil

½ an onion, finely chopped

500g lean mince

30ml water

1 tsp garlic granules

¼ tsp chilli flakes (optional)

3–4 drops Worcestershire sauce

1 tsp tomato purée

2 tbsp soy sauce

3 cherry tomatoes, chopped

1–2 gherkins, chopped

Salt to taste

3 slices American cheese
singles, torn

To build the taco:

4–6 taco shells

Iceberg lettuce, shredded

Cheddar cheese, grated

1 Grab a wok or high-sided pan and fry off the onion with a spray of oil until translucent, then add in the mince with the water (this will stop it from clumping together and keep it fine). Brown the meat, stirring regularly to let it cook evenly.

2 When the mince is cooked through, add in the garlic granules and chilli flakes, the Worcestershire sauce, tomato purée and soy sauce and mix well, allowing to cook for a further 2–3 minutes.

3 Add in your chopped tomatoes and gherkins and mix through, then add a pinch of salt and the cheese singles, stirring until these have melted in.

4 Heat the taco shells in the microwave for a few seconds, then spoon in some lettuce, a few heaped tablespoons of the cheesy mince mixture and a sprinkle of grated Cheddar on top.

Chicken Caesar
BURGER

This is one of my ultimate favourite burgers to throw on for a weekend fake make, with a side of Parmesan fries (see page 16). Crunchy, zingy and absolutely delicious! A take on the classic salad, making it more of a meal for the heartier appetite. You are going to love this one!

SERVES 2

30g panko breadcrumbs

½ tsp garlic powder

½ tsp smoked paprika

Salt to taste

2 chicken breasts

Low-calorie spray oil

For the bun seasoning:

1 tsp garlic powder

1 tsp mixed herbs

Salt to taste

2 wholemeal burger buns

To build the burger:

Iceberg lettuce, shredded

2–3 tbsp light Caesar dressing

Parmesan shavings

1 If not using an airfryer, preheat the oven to 220°C.

2 Mix the breadcrumbs in a bowl with the garlic powder, smoked paprika and salt to taste.

3 Slice the chicken breasts in half lengthways to get 4 pieces, removing the scaldy bits. Spritz with a little oil to dampen, dip into the breadcrumb mix and coat fully.

4 Spray the coated fillets with oil and pop in the airfryer at 190°C for 15 minutes or on a baking tray and into the preheated oven for 20–25 minutes until golden and crisp.

5 Next prepare your buns. Heat a large frying pan with a little spray of oil, and scatter in the garlic powder, mixed herbs and salt. Grab your buns and place them flat-side down, rubbing them around the pan to coat with the herbs for up to a minute, then toast under the grill.

6 When the buns are ready, layer with some iceberg lettuce, a piece of crispy chicken, a drizzle of Caesar dressing, a sprinkle of Parmesan, then another piece of crispy chicken. Finish with the top bun.

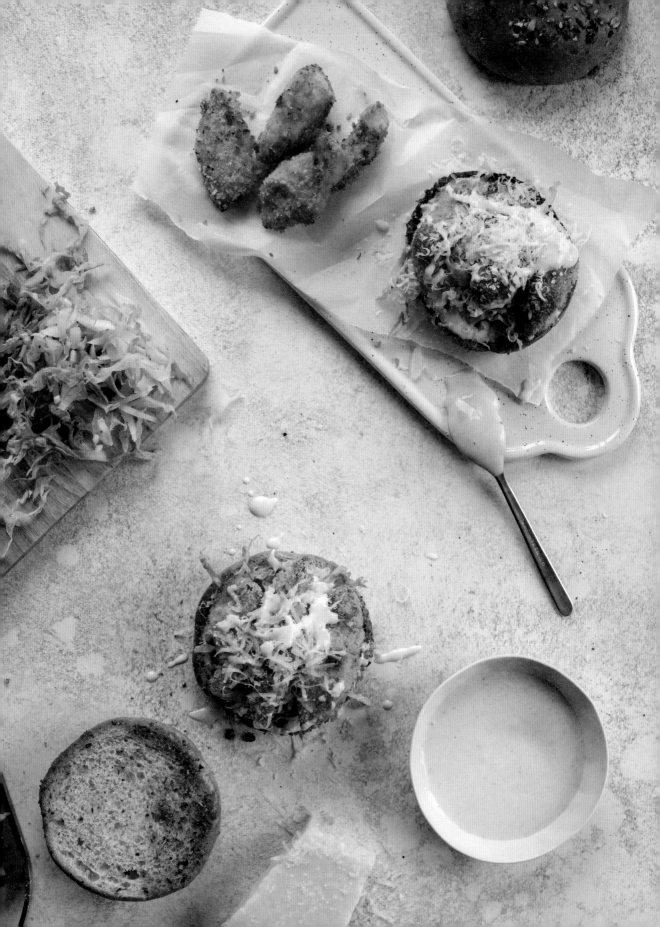

Pork Tenderloin
BURGER

One of our favourite things to do is to watch American fast-food shows, see what they are cooking and eating, then try to create the ones we like the look of but with our trademark healthier spin. This is one that we wanted to try and the version we made didn't disappoint!

SERVES 2

2 pork loin medallions, trimmed of excess fat
2 eggs
30g panko breadcrumbs
1 tbsp lemon pepper
Low-calorie spray oil

To build the buger:

2 wholemeal burger buns
2 tbsp lighter than light mayo
Iceberg lettuce, shredded
2 slices American cheese
1 gherkin, sliced

1 Preheat your oven to 220°C.

2 Start by butterflying your medallions: slice through the middle, but not completely, then open up into a 'butterfly' shape. Place them between two pieces of baking paper and give them a good wallop with a rolling pin to flatten them out as thin as you can. If you have a tenderiser, give them a few bangs of that too.

3 Get two bowls, whisk the eggs in one and mix the panko and lemon pepper in the other one.

4 Dip the medallions into the egg then into in the panko, making sure each one is completely covered with the seasoned crumbs.

5 Pop on to a baking sheet and cook in the oven for 25 minutes with a spray of oil, turning halfway through, or pop in the airfryer at 190°C for 15 minutes with a spray of oil turning halfway through.

6 Toast your buns, then layer up with mayo, lettuce, crispy pork medallions, cheese and pickles. Devour!

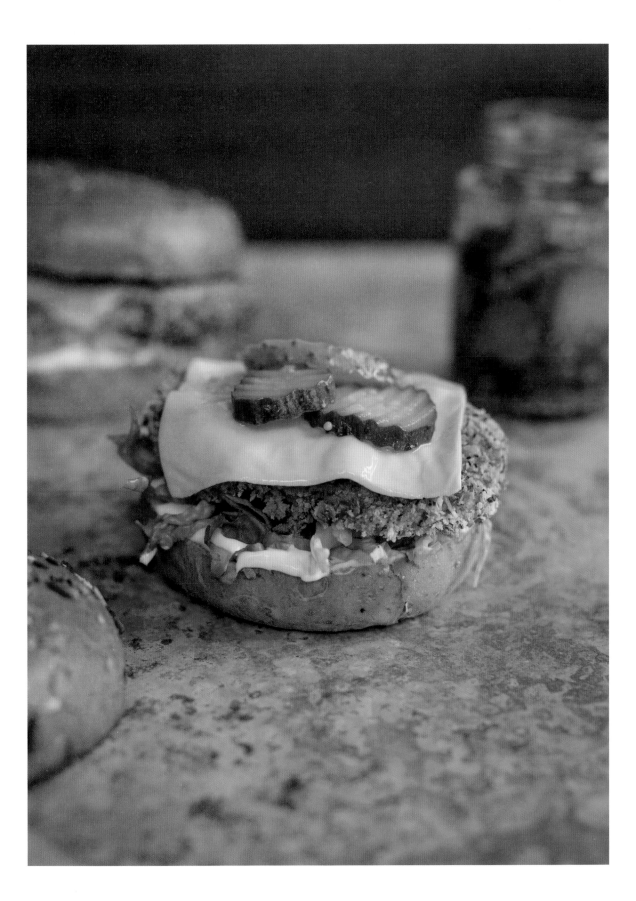

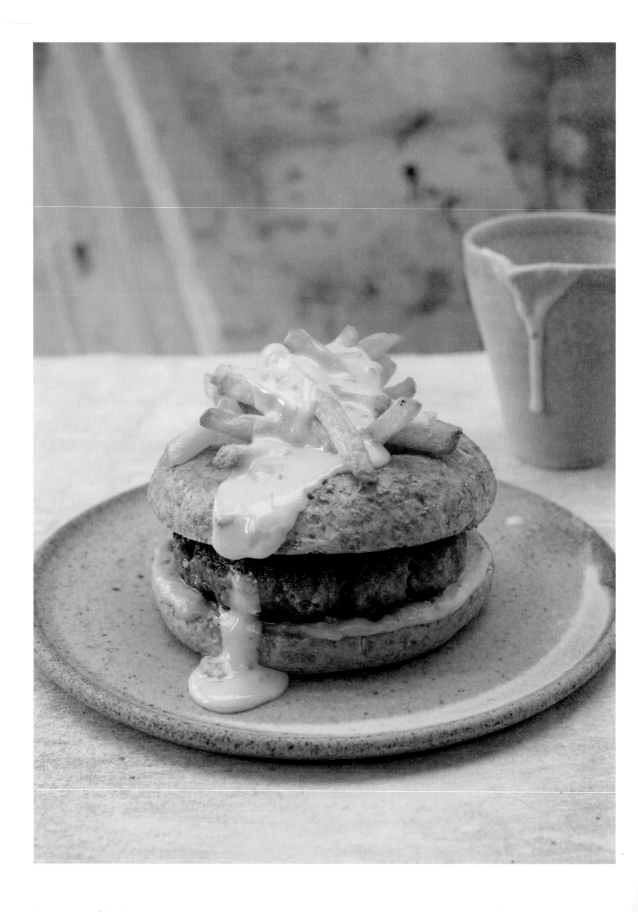

Volcano
BURGER

We don't watch much TV, but when we do, we watch food programmes. If we aren't cooking, we are watching other people cooking! One day we were watching a show and they made a 'fondue' burger and I swear, I nearly shed a tear. It was everything I could want from a burger – a burger, fries and cheese sauce. So, I legged it to the shops, because I knew I could make this bad boy in a less calorific way. That day, the volcano burger was born.

SERVES 4

1 kg potatoes

Low-calorie spray oil

500g lean mince

Salt and pepper to taste

2 tbsp hot sauce (more if you love it like we do)

3 light cheese slices, torn

100ml water

4–5 red jalapeño slices, from a jar

4 wholemeal bagel slims

1 Start by making your fries (see Perfect Chips, page 6).

2 Grab a big bowl, put in your mince and season with the salt, pepper and hot sauce.

3 Make 4 burger patties with the mince, as flat as you can. Using a shot glass or a small cookie cutter, cut a hole in the middle of each.

4 Heat a pan on a medium heat and cook the patties, turning after 5–7 minutes, until cooked through and nice and crusty on each side.

5 To make the lava, put the cheese slices and water in a little pot over a medium heat, let the mixture blend until smooth and silky, then add the jalapeño slices to make it nacho style.

6 Halve your bagels and toast them, then start to build your volcano burgers. So, bagel, burger patty, bagel and stuff the hole in the middle with as many fries as you can.

7 Next drizzle the nacho cheesy sauce all over the top like molten lava ... UNREAL. Grab your volcano burger with both hands and say a prayer!

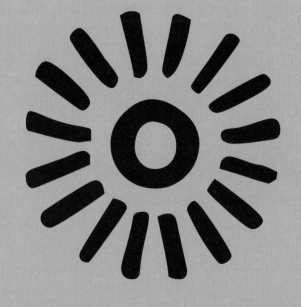

FOOD
TRUCK
EATS

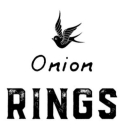

Onion
RINGS

The legend that is the onion ring is a staple of any good takeaway order. This is a super-quick recipe that delivers a banging end result. Awesome served with some dip or great to pop on top of a burger.

SERVES 2

2 large onions, sliced into thick circles

120g plain flour

350ml sparkling water

2 tsp lemon pepper

1 tsp garlic granules

1 tsp Cajun seasoning

Salt and pepper to taste

350ml rapeseed oil

1 Separate your onion slices into rings and place to one side while you get on with the batter.

2 Grab a mixing bowl and add in your flour followed by three-quarters of the sparkling water. Grab a whisk and whisk it all together, getting rid of any lumps. Gradually add the rest of the water, whisking as you go. You want a nice thick consistency to the batter – not watery – so add the water slowly and stop if the batter seems to be thick enough.

3 At this point add your lemon pepper, garlic granules, Cajun seasoning and salt and pepper to the batter, and whisk everything together.

4 Grab a wok or similar high-sided pan and add in your oil. What I do is slightly tilt the wok to the side, making a small pool of oil, and then I pop the wok on a medium heat. Once it's nice and hot, get an onion ring, dip it into the batter, shaking off any excess, then straight into the oil. Give it around a minute, then use a chopstick or tongs to flip the onion ring over and repeat on the other side until lovely and golden. Shake off the excess oil and place on a plate while you make the rest.

5 Add a sprinkle of salt, then serve up and enjoy.

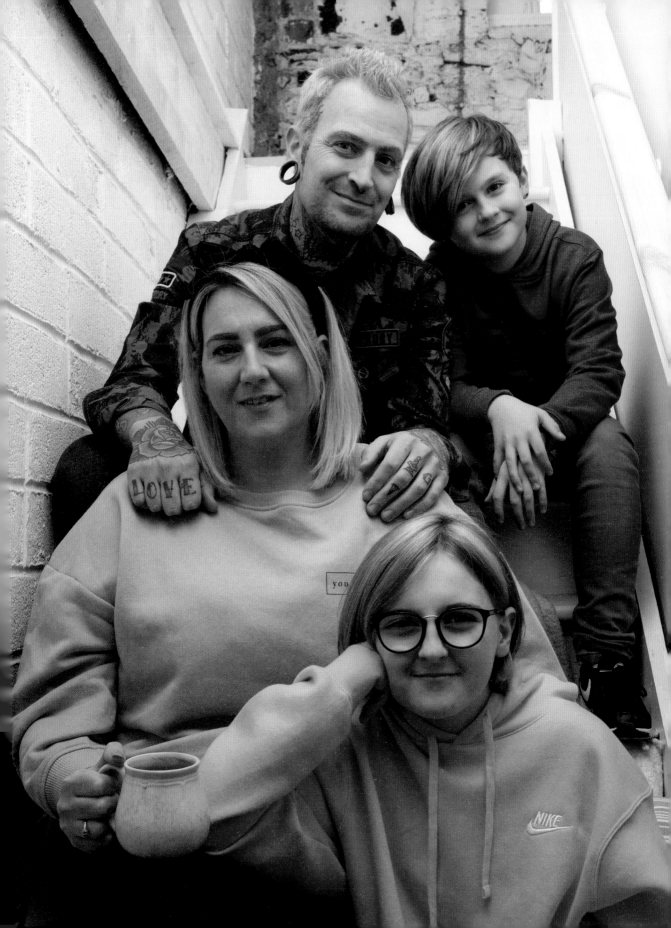

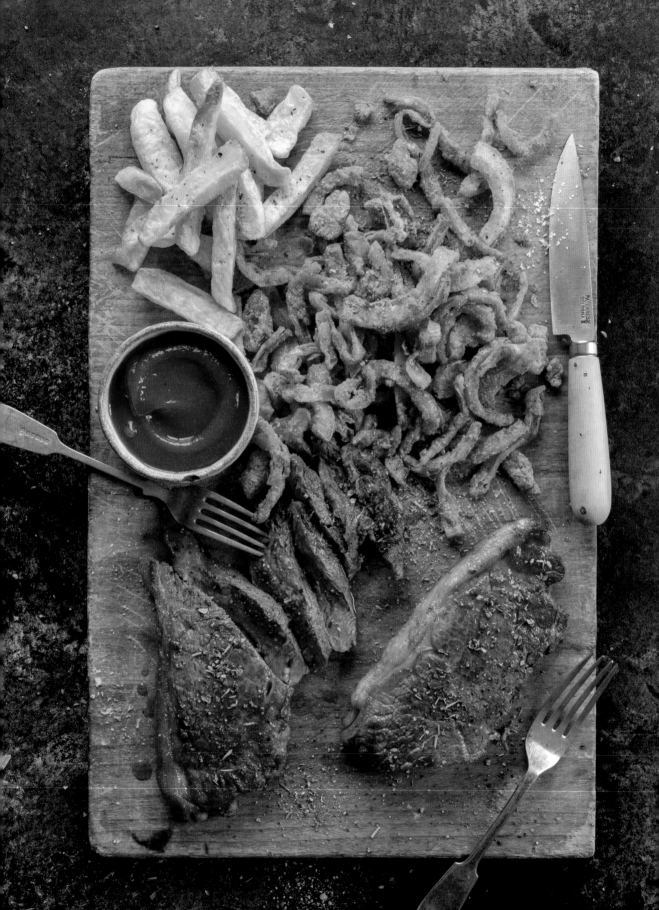

✳
Airfryer
CRISPY ONIONS

Every time I make steak, I just have to have crispy onions on the side. These are super quick to make and are absolutely gorgeous. They're great as a side and even better as a filler for a sambo or burger.

SERVES 2

2 yellow onions, peeled and sliced into strips

1 egg

3 tbsp cornflour

1 tsp smoked paprika

1 tsp garlic powder

low-calorie spray oil

salt, to taste

1 Beat your egg in a bowl. In a separate bowl, mix together the cornflour, paprika and garlic powder.

2 First dip your onion strips into the egg and then into the cornflour mix, getting them nice and coated.

3 Give them a couple of sprays of low-calorie spray oil and pop them into the airfryer for around 8 minutes at 180°C, giving them a good shake halfway through.

4 When they're ready, sprinkle them with salt and serve.

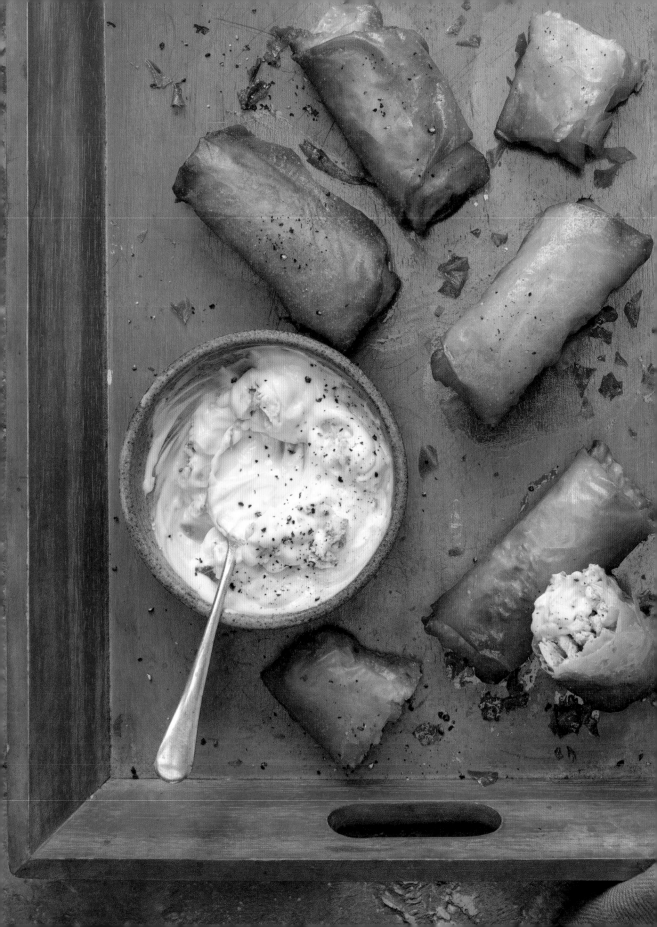

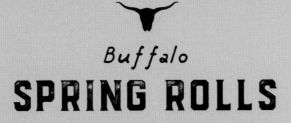

Buffalo
SPRING ROLLS

Tangy, cheesy with a little kick of spice and a gorgeous, crunchy outside, change up the tradition of the spring roll and get creative with these masso versions! If you think it, you can make it and this one is perfect for all you buffalo spice lovers.

SERVES 4

2 chicken breasts, cooked and shredded (see Easy Shredded Chicken recipe, page 158)

250ml buffalo hot sauce

30g Cheddar cheese, grated

Filo pastry or 4 spring roll wrappers (available from Asian supermarkets)

35g blue cheese

1 scallion, finely sliced

8 cherry tomatoes, chopped

Caesar dressing

Low-calorie spray oil

1 If not using an airfryer, preheat your oven to 200°C.

2 Put the shredded chicken in a warm pan and add the hot sauce, mix it through until the chicken is coated, then add in the Cheddar cheese. Allow the cheese to melt in.

3 Lay out the filo pastry and cut each piece in half until you have 4 squares. Otherwise lay out 4 wrappers.

4 With one of the corners facing you, put 2 tablespoons of the mixture in a line across the middle of the pastry, making sure not to bring it to the edges, sprinkle a little blue cheese on top and add some scallion, tomato and a drizzle of Caesar dressing.

5 Bring the corner facing you over the top of the mixture and tuck it under the filling, then bring in the right and left corners towards the centre and continue to roll until it's nice and tight. Repeat the process with the remaining wrappers. Now we want to crisp them up on the outside. I usually pop the rolls in the airfryer with a light spray of oil for 6–7 minutes at 180°C until golden brown (or you can pop them in the preheated oven for 15 minutes).

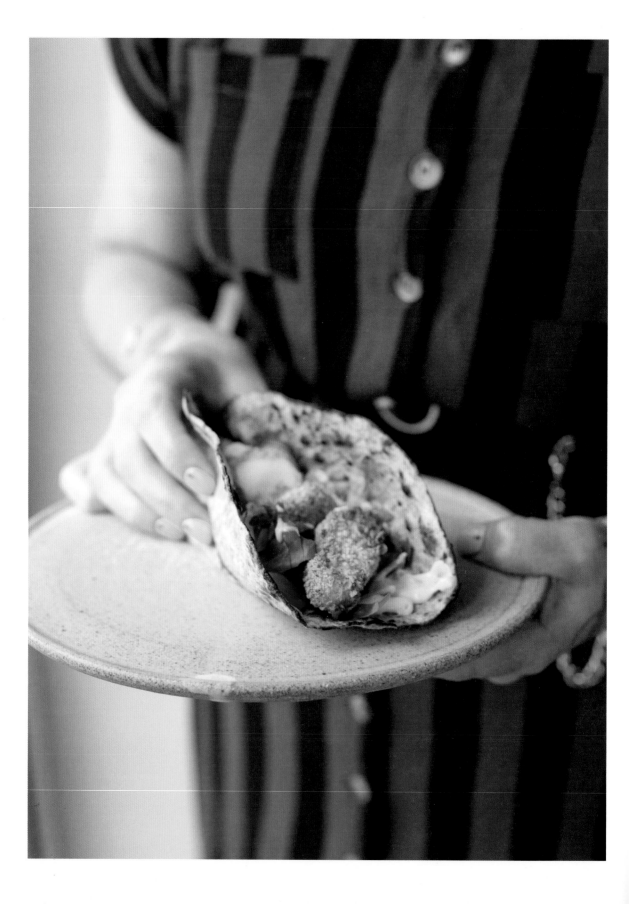

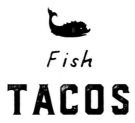

Fish

TACOS

These super-easy fish tacos are a deadly family meal. We use cod or haddock as it's firmer but you can use whatever fish you prefer. You can pan fry the fish too if you would prefer it not to be crispy, but you know us, the crispier the better. The zingy sauce is absolutely massive drizzled over the top. Jaysus I think I'll go and make some now, I'm making myself hungry!

SERVES 4

40g panko breadcrumbs

1 tsp smoked paprika

1 tsp garlic granules

Salt and pepper to taste

1 egg

300g fresh cod or haddock fillets, cut into goujons

6–7 sprays of rapeseed oil

For the sauce:

3 tbsp lighter than light mayo

1 tsp yellow American mustard

1 pickled gherkin, finely chopped

1 tsp pickle juice from the gherkin jar

1 garlic clove, finely minced

Juice of ½ a lime

To build the tacos:

4–6 small wholemeal wraps

Shredded lettuce

1 red onion, halved then finely sliced into half moons

1 large tomato, diced

3–4 tbsp tinned sweetcorn

1 radish, finely sliced

Fresh coriander (if it's for you)

1 Preheat the oven to 200°C.

2 Lash the panko, smoked paprika and garlic granules, along with the salt and pepper, into a bowl and mix well.

3 Beat the egg in a separate bowl, then dip the goujons first into the egg, then into the spice mix, making sure they are coated evenly.

4 Spray a baking tray with a little oil and evenly lay out the coated pieces of fish on it. Pop in the preheated oven and cook for 15–20 minutes, turning and spraying with a little oil halfway through, until the coating is golden and brown.

5 To make the sauce, mix all the ingredients in a small ramekin and put to one side.

6 Heat the wraps on a dry pan until soft or pop in the microwave for 20 seconds, then lash on the lettuce, onion, tomato and cooked fish goujons. Finish by shaking over some sweetcorn, drizzle over the sauce, and garnish with some radish and optional coriander.

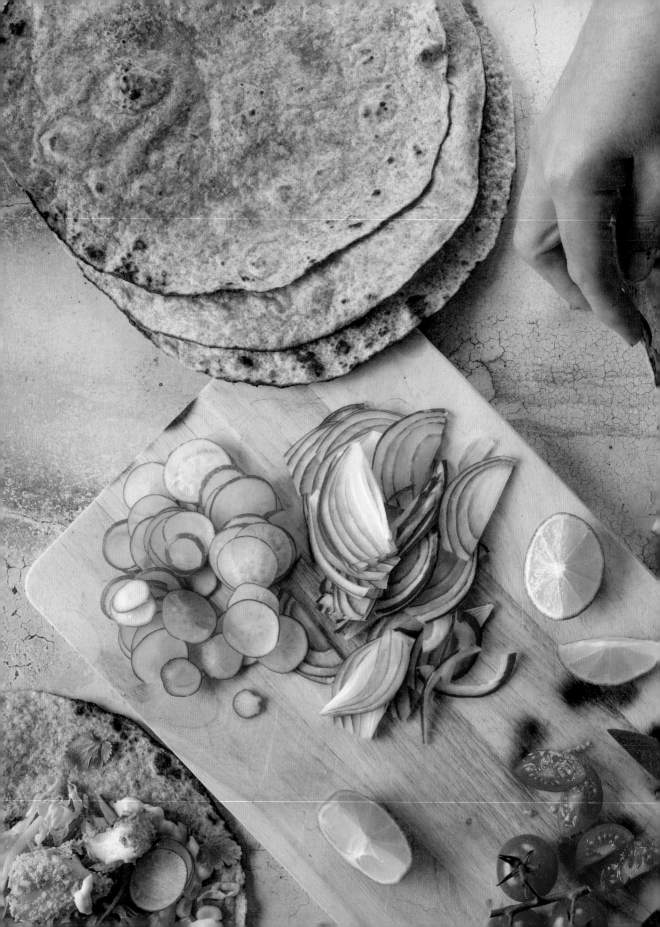

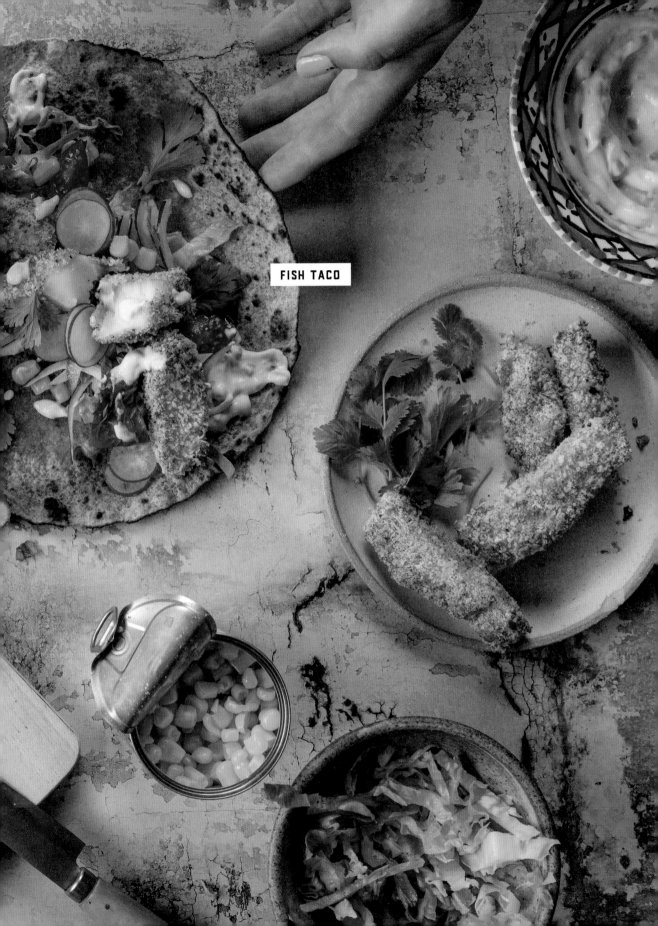

FISH TACO

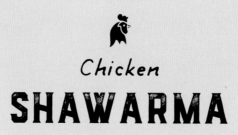

Chicken
SHAWARMA

This used to be my go-to in the takeaway, loaded with a rake of sauce after a few drinks, but now I can make a healthier version in my gaff and have it anytime I want! It's super straightforward and with all the herbs and spices available now in your local supermarket it's never been easier to recreate mega dishes like this. If you can't find shawarma spice made up it's a doddle to create at home. Just remember you need to marinate the chicken overnight so you'll need to do this the night before you want to eat it.

SERVES 6

8 chicken thigh fillets, all visible fat removed

For the shawarma spice marinade:

1 tbsp ground cumin

1 tsp turmeric

2 tsp smoked paprika

½ tsp ground cardamom

1 tsp ground coriander

½ tsp ground ginger

200ml water

To serve:

6 wholemeal pittas, warmed

Iceberg lettuce, shredded

1 red onion, sliced

A drizzle of garlic sauce

1 Preheat your oven to 220°C.

2 Start by marinating the chicken. Mix the spices with the water in a large bowl. Add in the chicken thighs and massage in the spices, making sure they are completely covered. Cover with clingfilm and pop into the fridge overnight.

3 To cook, you will need to stick the chicken on skewers, which is easy to do! We have a kebab spike, but you can make a DIY version at home. Get a baking tray, cut a large onion or potato in half, stick two bamboo skewers beside each other into one half of the potato or onion and then layer up the chicken piece by piece. Once it's been layered up, pop into the oven for 40 minutes until golden and brown.

4 Remove and allow to stand for 10 minutes and then slice those babies up. Serve in warm pittas with lettuce and red onion and drizzle on some garlic sauce.

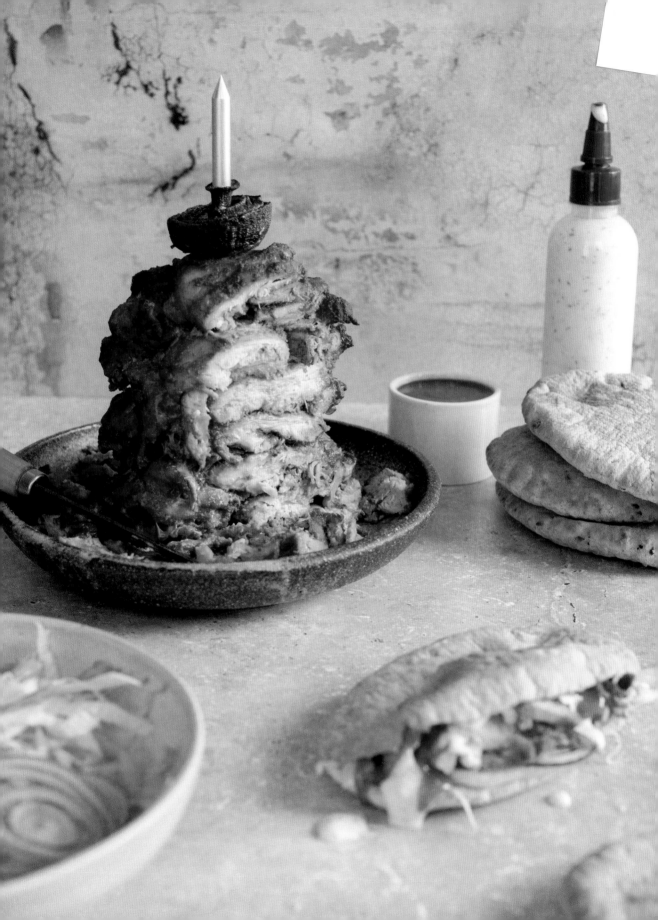

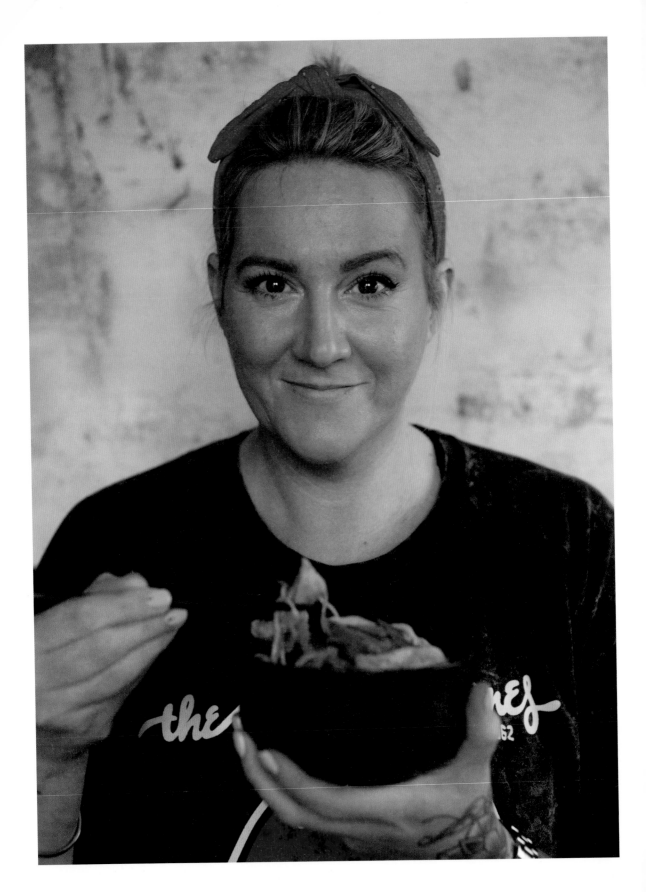

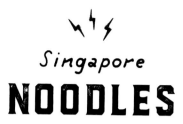

Singapore

NOODLES

A super-cool recipe with a little kick. I love extra-fine noodles and this is a great recipe to use them in. Packed full of fresh veggies and spicy, fragrant flavours, you will love this!

SERVES 2

200g fine egg noodles

Low-calorie spray oil

1 onion, finely sliced

1 carrot, julienned or grated

1 red pepper, deseeded and sliced

1 green pepper, deseeded and sliced

2 chicken breasts, boiled and shredded (see page 158)

2 tbsp soy sauce

1 tbsp mild curry powder

½ tsp garlic granules

½ tsp turmeric

½ tsp ground ginger

¼ tsp chilli flakes (more if you like a good kick)

2 scallions, finely sliced

1 Start with the noodles – pop them into a bowl or pan, pour over some boiling water and let them soften for the amount of time it says on the packet.

2 Heat a wok with a little oil and stir-fry the onion, carrot and peppers.

3 Add in the shredded chicken, then the soy sauce, curry powder, garlic granules, turmeric, ginger and chilli flakes, stirring well to coat the chicken and veg in the spices. Add in the drained noodles and stir to heat through. Finish by scattering over the sliced scallions.

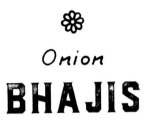

Onion
BHAJIS

These were always a favourite of mine when it came to getting an Indian takeaway – we always ordered some onion bhajis for a starter. I knew I wanted to recreate them at home and have a healthier take than the deep-fried ones you would usually get from a restaurant, and these ones are the business.

SERVES 8

60g plain flour

1 tsp garlic granules

1 tsp turmeric

1 tsp ground cumin

1 tsp garam masala

½ tsp chilli flakes

100ml water

1 yellow onion halved and sliced

1 red onion, halved and sliced

1 jalapeño pepper, deseeded and diced (optional)

Low-calorie spray oil

1 If not using an airfryer, preheat the oven to 180°C.

2 Put your flour and spices in a mixing bowl and gradually stir in the water, mixing everything together until smooth – you want to take out any lumps and have a nice even consistency.

3 Now here comes the messy part – add your onions and jalapenos into the spicy mix, and using your hands, get stuck in and mix everything together.

4 Lay out some baking paper on the counter beside you, form 8 equal portions and place them on it. Don't panic, they seem like they're gonna fall apart but they won't.

5 Now, the way I cook these is to start them on the pan and then move to the airfryer or oven. So get your pan ready, give it a few sprays of oil and place on a medium heat. Using a fish slice, carefully scoop the bhajis onto the pan, giving them a minute or two on each side, which will solidify them. Then transfer to a baking tray and pop into the preheated oven, or into your airfryer at 180°C for around 6 minutes until crisp and golden, turning them halfway through.

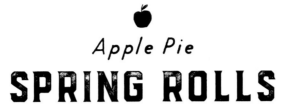

Apple Pie
SPRING ROLLS

Okay, so these are just unreal and super-simple to make, kind of a takeaway-style hot apple pie vibe but without the deep fryer and all the oil. Super-handy to prepare in advance and then just pop in the oven or airfryer while you are eating dinner and they'll be nice and hot for dessert! Absolute perfection!

SERVES 4

4–5 eating apples, peeled and chopped into small cubes

1 tsp ground cinnamon

1 tbsp granulated sweetener (plus extra for dusting)

4 spring roll wrappers (available from Asian supermarkets)

Low-calorie spray oil

1 If not using an airfryer, preheat the oven to 200°C.

2 Grab a saucepan and put in the apples, cinnamon and sweetener. Cook on a medium heat for 10–15 minutes, giving the odd stir, until the apples have softened. Taste and add more cinnamon or sweetener if you think it needs it.

3 Lay out a spring roll wrapper so it's in a diamond shape (one point facing towards you). Dollop 2–3 tablespoons of the apple filling in a line across the centre, then you need to wrap it up.

4 Bring the corner pointing towards you up over the filling, then fold over the left and the right corner to meet in the middle, then roll it up until you have a spring roll shape. Repeat with the remaining wrappers.

5 Pop them into the airfryer at 180°C with a little spray of oil for 10–12 minutes, or pop on a baking tray lined with greaseproof paper and cook in the preheated oven for 20 minutes, turning halfway through, until golden and crisp.

6 Serve with a dusting of sweetener and a dollop of cream if you're a mad thing!

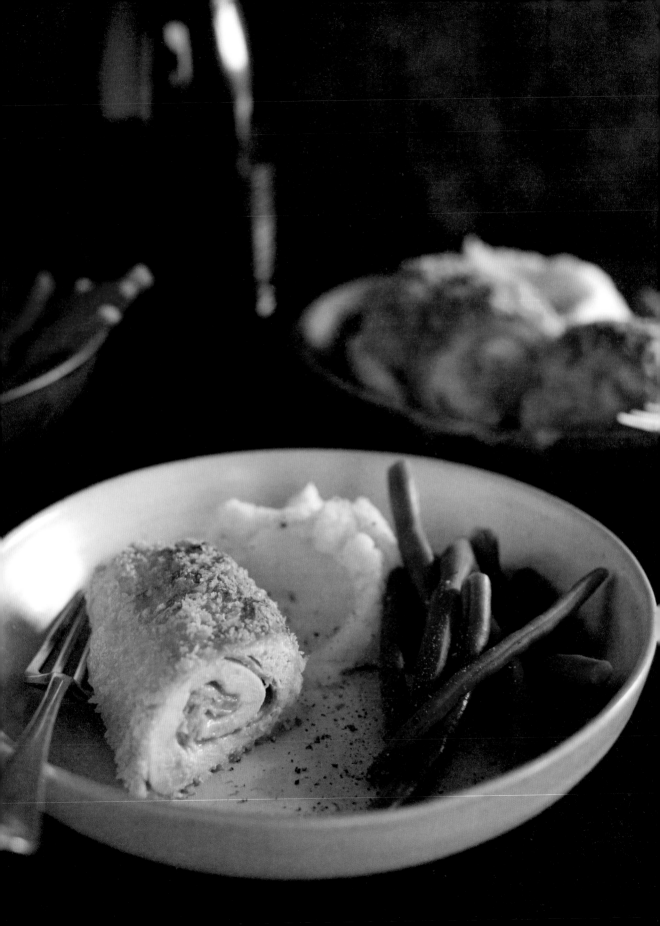

★ ★ ★

Chicken
CORDON BLEU

I was 17 years old when I first had this dish and I still remember it like it was yesterday. We used to go to a hotel on the Captain's Hill in Leixlip and this was one of their specialities. I had to ask what it was as I'd never heard of it before but I've loved it ever since and it always brings back great family-time memories. Chicken Cordon Bleu is a classic chicken dish stuffed with cheese and ham, then coated in a crispy crumb and cooked so the cheese is all melty and delicious inside.

SERVES 2

2 chicken breasts
2 slices Cheddar cheese
2 slices carved ham

For the coating:

1 egg
30g panko breadcrumbs
3 tbsp Grana Padano cheese, grated
Low-calorie spray oil

1 If not using an airfryer, preheat the oven to 220°C.

2 Start by butterflying the chicken breasts (see page 36), then lay them out on some baking paper, cover with cling film and give them a little bash with a rolling pin to flatten them out.

3 Then pop a slice of the cheddar and ham in the middle of each piece of chicken and roll it up tight. Pop a toothpick in to secure the edges and prevent the ham and cheese from coming out. You can also or wrap the parcels tightly in cling film and pop in the fridge for a few hours to firm them up and hold their shape when you remove it.

4 Now we can get on with the coating. Get two bowls, whisk the egg in one and put the panko and grated Grana Padano in the other one.

5 Dip the chicken parcels first in the egg, then in the panko mix, making sure they are well coated.

6 Pop in the airfryer for 15–20 mins at 190°C until golden and crisp or pop on a baking sheet and into the preheated oven for 25 minutes.

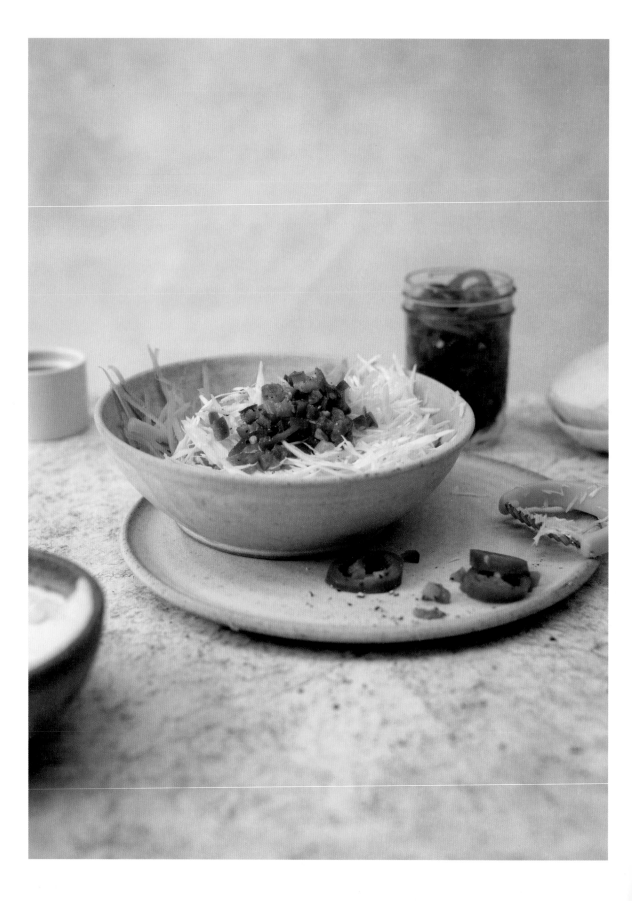

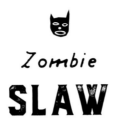

Zombie

SLAW

'Zombie' is the perfect name for this slaw with an added kick. It goes great with burgers, salads, toasties and more. Quick and simple to make.

SERVES 6

½ a white cabbage, finely chopped

3 carrots, grated

25g jarred jalapeños, chopped (use more or less depending on how hot you like it)

5 tbsp light mayonnaise

5 tbsp hot sauce (your preferred brand)

Freshly ground black pepper

Put the cabbage, carrot, and chopped jalapeños in a mixing bowl. Add in the mayo, hot sauce, and a sprinkle of pepper. Mix thoroughly together, ensuring everything is coated.

♥

Garlic and Chilli
PIL PIL PRAWNS

Here's a great quick little starter for you, really easy to make and takes no time at all. Serve with some crusty bread on the side to mop up the juices.

SERVES 2

3 tbsp olive oil

2 garlic cloves, finely sliced

1 fresh red chilli, deseeded and sliced

250g fresh prawns, cleaned and shelled

Salt and pepper to taste

½ tsp smoked paprika

1 tbsp fresh parsley, chopped

1 Grab a pan (preferably a small one), get your oil in and put on a medium heat. Get it nice and hot then add in the garlic and chilli, stirring around for around 30 seconds until the garlic is softening.

2 Add in the prawns and allow to cook until pink, stirring regularly, and then serve up garnished with some salt, pepper and a sprinkle of smoked paprika and fresh parsley.

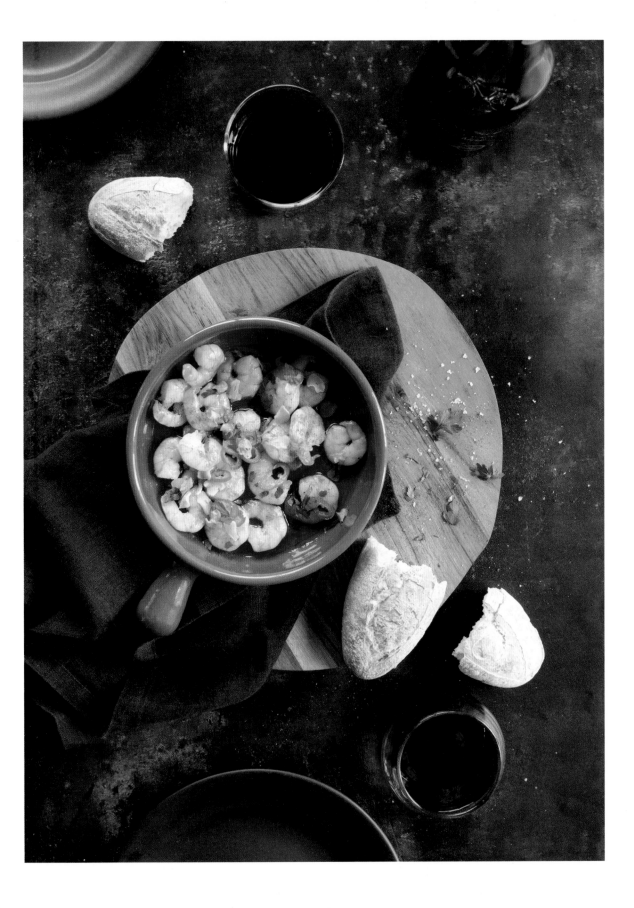

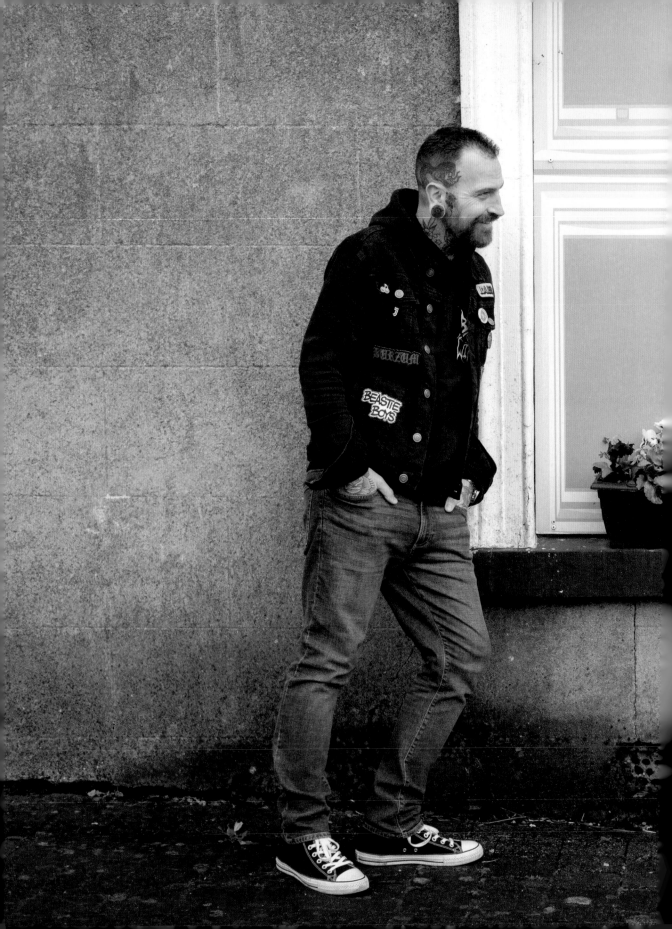

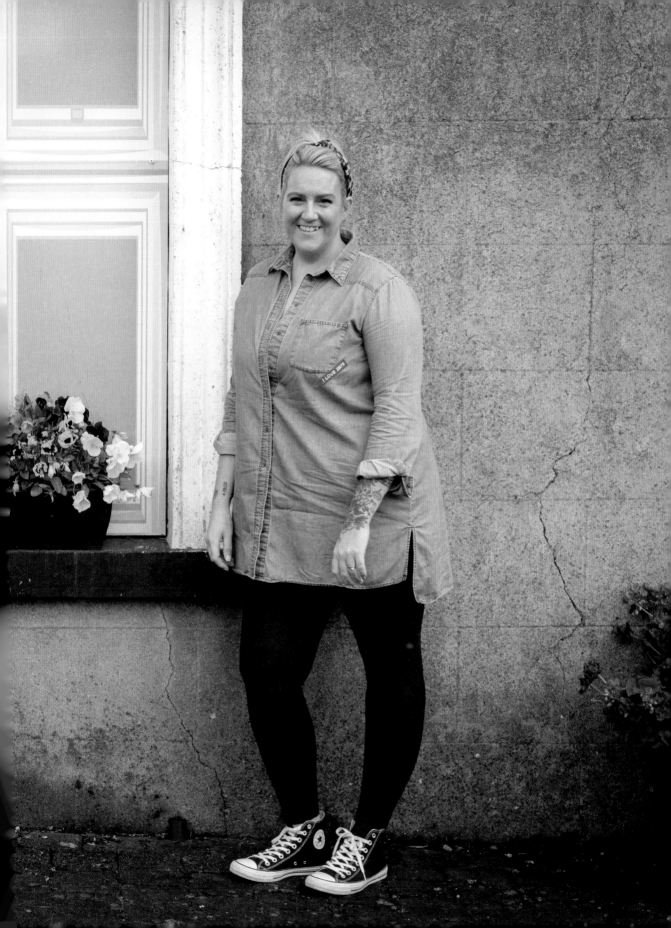

✳
Baked Jalapeño
POPPERS

Jalapeño poppers are hollowed-out chillies stuffed with creamy cream cheese and Cheddar, topped with smoky bacon bits and breadcrumbs, then baked to perfection. They make the perfect starter or nibble and will give you a nice spicy kick.

SERVES 4-5

4 smoked bacon medallions

10 fresh jalapeño chillies

150g light cream cheese

40g Cheddar cheese, grated

15g panko breadcrumbs

1 tbsp Grana Padano cheese, grated

1 tbsp chopped chives

1 Preheat your oven to 200°C.

2 First pop the bacon under the grill, cook until golden and crisp, chop finely, and set aside.

3 Then start with one whole chilli and slice in half lengthways. Use the handle of a teaspoon to scrape out the seeds and membrane, then repeat until all the chillies are halved and deseeded. Make sure you wash your hands after you've handled the chilli seeds!

4 In a bowl, mix the light cream cheese with the Cheddar, then carefully fill the chilli 'boats'.

5 In another bowl, mix the panko with the Grana Padano and sprinkle the mixture over each filled chilli boat.

6 Lay out the filled jalapeños (carefully spaced out) on a baking sheet lined with greaseproof paper, and pop in the preheated oven for 10–12 minutes until they start to char and the cheese is lovely and melty.

7 Remove and sprinkle with the chopped bacon and chives.

Slow Cooker
SHREDDED BEEF

I'm not a one-trick pony, I can actually manage to use another appliance that isn't an airfryer lol ... well, just about! The slow cooker is actually a little lifesaver when you are short on time or have a busy lifestyle but want loads of flavour and a deadly dinner. You can prep it all in advance, lash it on in the morning and come home to something wonderful. The beef in this will shred like butter and you'll be lucky if you don't eat it all from the crockpot with a spoon!

SERVES 4-6

800g lean diced beef

400ml passata

4 tbsp hot sauce

1 tsp garlic granules

½ tsp Worcestershire sauce

½ tsp chilli powder

½ tsp smoked paprika

1 beef stock pot, dissolved in 200ml boiling water

1 tbsp apple cider vinegar

1 tsp brown sugar

1 Start by searing the beef in a hot pan, this will give the meat a nice brown coating and add extra flavour to your sauce during the cooking process.

2 Put the beef in the slow cooker and add the passata first, then just lob everything else in – seriously, so, so easy! When you have all your ingredients in the pot give it a good stir to blend everything together.

3 Pop it on low for 8 hours or high for 4 hours and then go about your day as normal. When the time is up, use two forks to shred up the beef. It should be super-tender and fall apart nicely.

4 You can serve it in wraps, tacos, loaded on top of fries, with nachos or piled into a baked potato – masso!

Mexican

STREET CORN

We all love Mexican food in the Dish house; one of Ben's favourites is the classic burrito. I love a good starter before a weekend Mexican feast and corn on the cob was one I'd do every now and then – but how can you make corn on the cob a little more adventurous and exciting? Well, you make Mexican Street Corn!

SERVES 4

8 frozen mini ears of corn

4 tbsp lighter than light mayo

1 tsp cayenne pepper

1 tsp hot sauce

A handful of fresh coriander, finely chopped

1 lime

Salt and pepper to taste

Low-calorie spray oil

20g mozzarella cheese, grated

1 Start by cooking your corn in boiling water for around 10 minutes.

2 While your corn is on the boil, put the mayo, cayenne pepper, hot sauce and coriander into a bowl. Squeeze over half the lime, add some salt and pepper, then mix everything together and put to one side.

3 Remove your corn from the pot using tongs and shake off any excess water. Give them a light spray of oil and pop into the airfryer for 4–5 minutes at 180°C, or place under a grill on a medium to high heat for the same time, turning halfway through, until golden.

4 Get your corn and lightly spread your mixture lengthways on top, finishing with a sprinkle of mozzarella. Pop under the grill for 60 seconds or so, remove, squeeze over the remaining half lime, and serve.

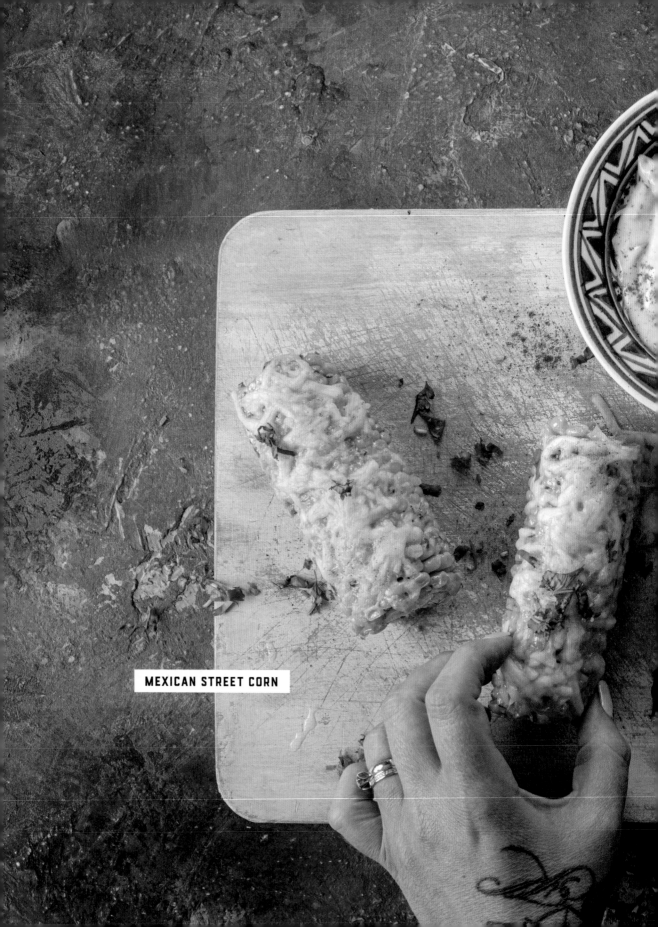

MEXICAN STREET CORN

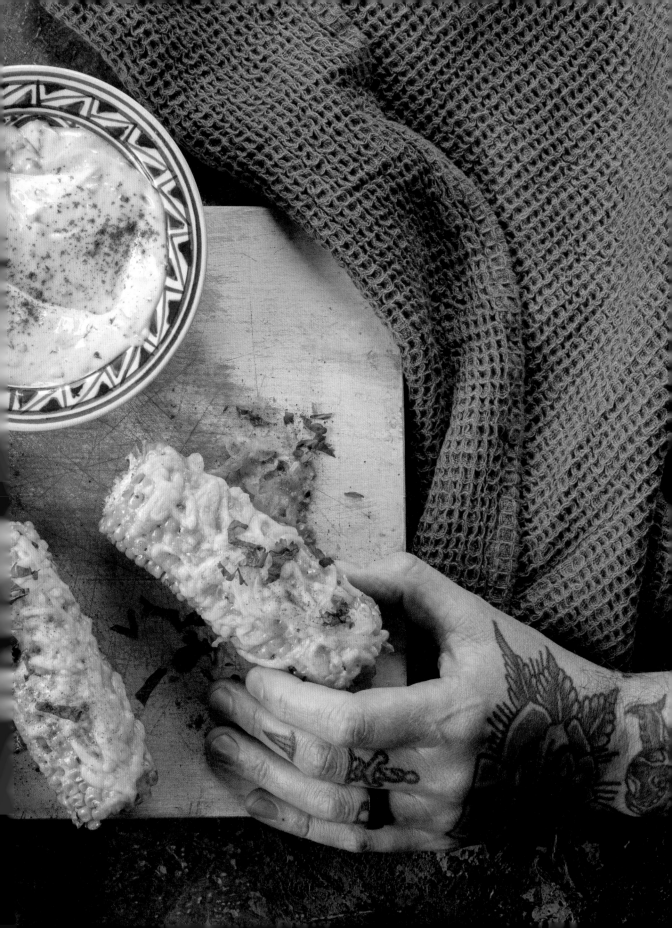

Crispy

COURGETTE FRIES

These make a tasty change from chips and they give you a bang of one of your five a day!

SERVES 2

2 courgettes, each end sliced off and cut into chip-shaped pieces

1 tsp garlic powder

½ tsp paprika

Salt to taste

2 eggs

40g panko breadcrumbs

15g Grana Padano cheese, grated

Low-calorie spray oil

1 Preheat your oven to 220°C.

2 Dry off your courgette 'chips' in a clean tea towel, pop in a Ziplock bag with the garlic powder, paprika and a pinch of salt, and give a good shake to ensure that each piece is coated.

3 Grab two bowls, one for the wet mix and one for the dry. Beat the eggs in one bowl and mix the panko breadcrumbs and Grana Padano together in another.

4 Dip the chips into the egg and then into the panko mix, making sure each one is well coated in crumbs.

5 Lay them out on a baking tray with a spray of oil (or pop in the airfryer at 190°C), turning halfway through and respraying to keep them from burning and to allow the fries to brown and crisp up.

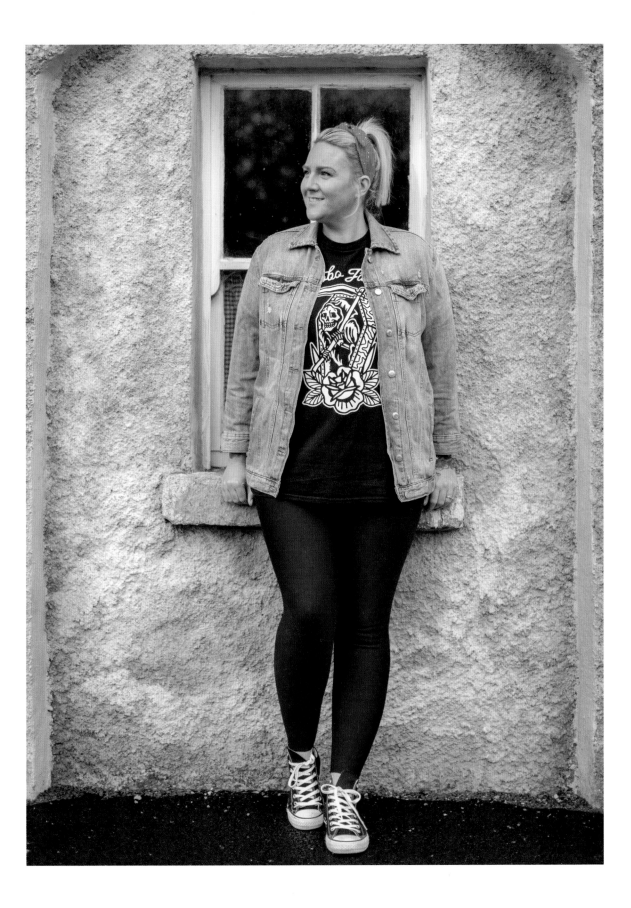

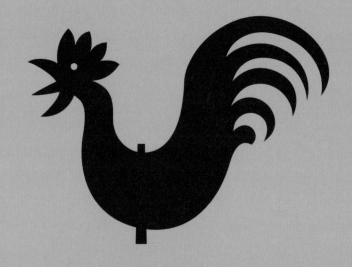

BANGING BREAKFAST AND BRUNCH

Brekkie
PIZZA WRAP

So I've mixed my love of the Irish breakfast with my love of pizza here to create an epic wrap to start your day off with. Great for a weekend brekkie or brunch, especially if you've had one or two drinks the night before. Quick and easy to make and one the whole family can enjoy.

SERVES 2

1 x 400g tin of baked beans

Low-calorie spray oil

4–5 slices of good-quality black pudding

6–8 mushrooms, sliced

8 cherry tomatoes, each cut into 4 slices

2 wholemeal wraps

15g Cheddar cheese, grated

15g mozzarella cheese, grated

Salt and pepper to taste

1 Throw your beans into a pot and get them heating.

2 Get your pudding cooking on a pan with a spray of oil, cook for a couple of minutes on each side then pop onto a plate, and use a fork to break it all up.

3 Give your mushrooms and tomatoes a couple of minutes on the pan too and get them cooked.

4 Next up, grab your wraps and spoon the hot beans onto them, covering the bases. Follow that up with the two cheeses and cooked veg, then sprinkle the crumbled pudding evenly over.

5 Pop the wraps under the grill for a couple of minutes to get the cheese melted, and season with some salt and pepper. You can slice like a pizza, or if you're like me roll them up and eat like a wrap. Enjoy.

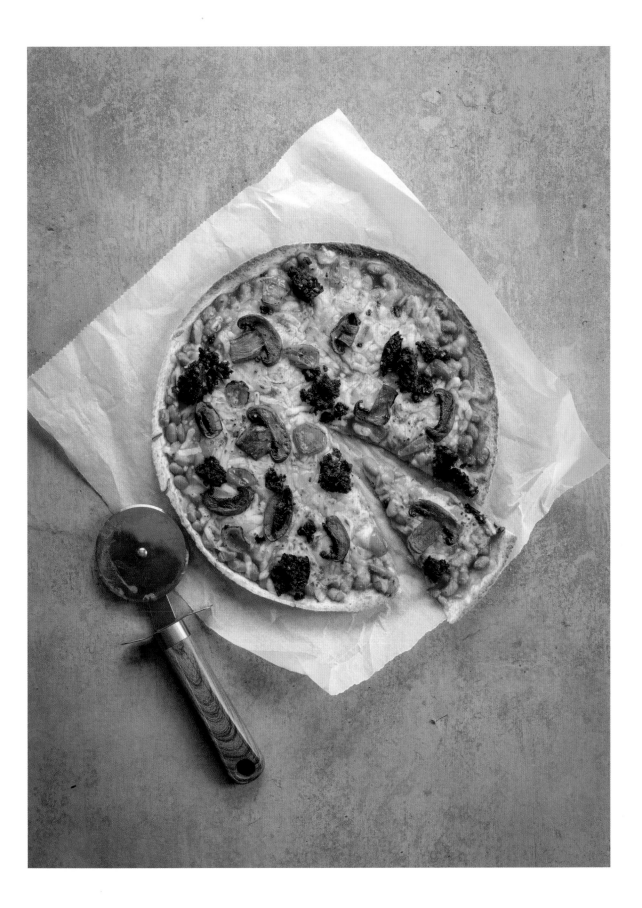

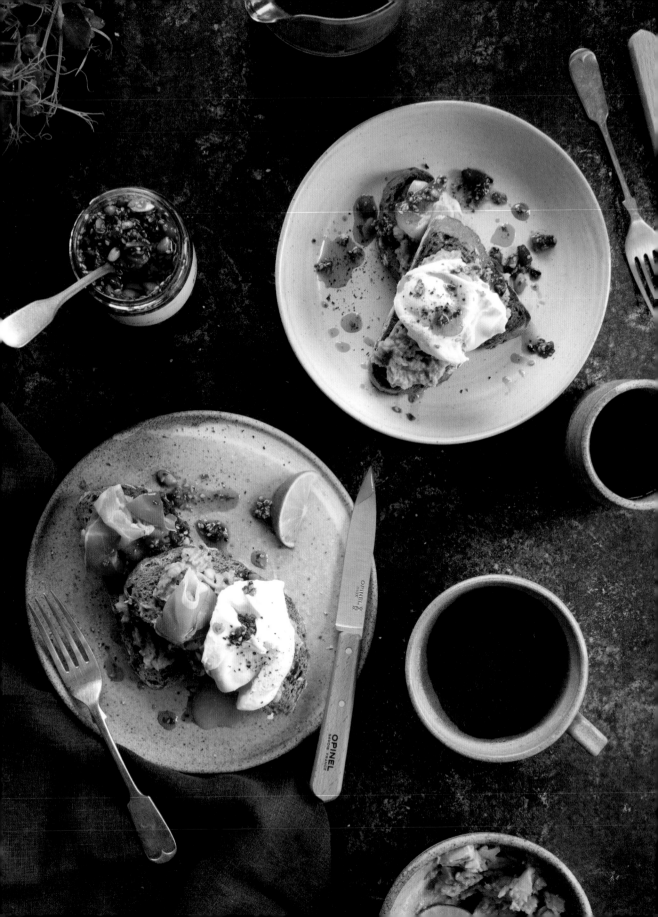

Posh

EGG AND TOAST

Here's another brunch favourite of mine, great for those lazy weekend mornings when you fancy something a little different. Quick and easy to prepare and bursting with flavour.

SERVES 1

½ a ripe avocado

½ a lime

Salt and pepper to taste

1 slice wholemeal bread

2 eggs

2 slices prosciutto

1 tsp peanut rayu (available in most supermarkets)

1 Grab your avocado and scoop the flesh into a small bowl, squeeze your lime in, add a little salt and pepper then mash well with a fork. Once it's all mixed up place to one side.

2 Get your toast on and cook your eggs the way you fancy them – I usually vary between poached or fried for this dish.

3 Once your bread is toasted, spread your avocado mix evenly onto it followed by your prosciutto and eggs. Spoon a little rayu over and sprinkle with a little salt and pepper.

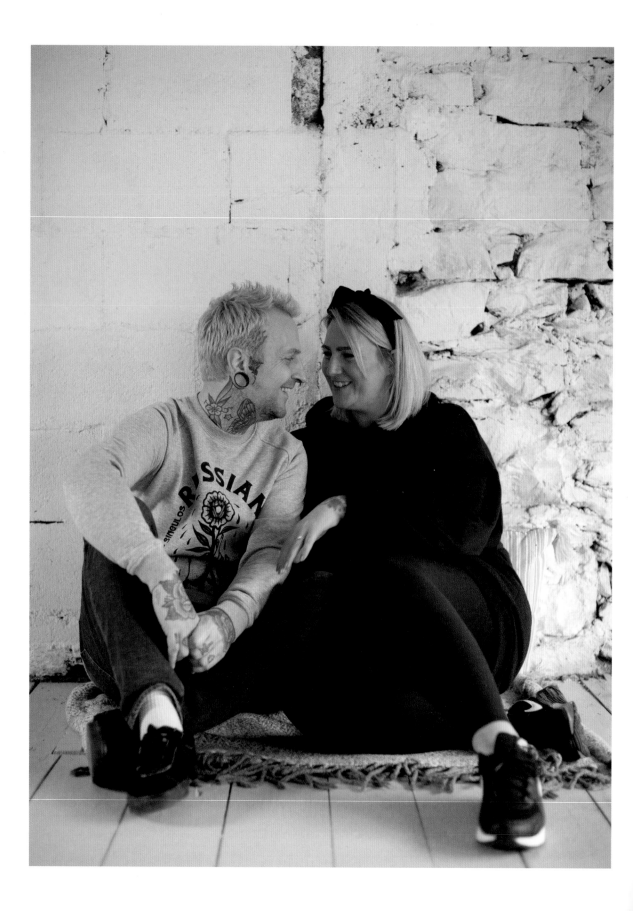

Parma Ham, Asparagus and
POACHED EGG

Crispy Parma ham is absolutely delicious but when you combine it with asparagus the taste is incredible. If that wasn't enough, add an oozy poached egg into the mix and your mind will be blown!

SERVES 2

12 fresh asparagus spears, woody ends cut off (2 per wrap, 3 wraps per person)

6 slices of Parma ham, excess fat removed

2 eggs

A dash of white vinegar

Salt and pepper to taste

1 Preheat the oven to 200°C.

2 Start by parboiling the asparagus for 2–3 minutes until the heavy crunch is gone, then drain.

3 Lay out the Parma ham slices, take two pieces of asparagus, place directly onto each slice and roll it up into a wrap. Repeat until you've used up all the asparagus.

4 Lay out the wraps on a baking sheet lined with parchment and cook for 10 minutes or until the ham has crisped up. Alternatively pop them in the airfryer at 180°C for 5–6 minutes.

5 To poach the eggs, crack the egg into a small ramekin. Add 3–4 inches of boiling water from the kettle to a small pot and pop it on a medium heat – you don't want the water to be bubbling because this will push the eggs around the pan and you'll lose some of the white. Add in the vinegar, and with the end of a wooden spoon stir the water in one direction until you have a little vortex in the centre.

6 Gently drop an egg in and the spinning will allow the white to form around the yolk. Spin the water a little around the edge of the pot then add the other egg. Cook for 3 minutes until the white is firmed up and remove to a plate, using a slotted spoon.

7 Serve the poached eggs on top of the crispy asparagus-Parma wraps and season with salt and pepper.

Peanut Butter

OVERNIGHT OATS

Skipping breakfast was always my downfall – if there wasn't anything 'handy' there I'd simply go without which would then lead me to eat rings around myself come lunchtime with crappy convenience food, because I was just 'too hungry' to cook anything. Having a handy grab-and-go brekkie ready from the night before will guarantee you won't go without all day and will get the engine started for the day ahead. This is very simple and so adaptable with so many different options – play around with flavours and ingredients and see what floats your boat. If you are not into cold oats you can give them a little zap in the microwave to warm the belly.

SERVES 1

40g porridge oats

100ml slimline milk

4 tbsp fat-free vanilla yoghurt

1 tsp chia seeds

1 tsp peanut butter powder (available from healthfood shops)

5–6 raspberries or 3–4 straw-berries

1 Mix all the ingredients in a Mason jar or lunchbox and seal or cover and leave in the fridge for a minimum of 3 hours, preferably overnight.

2 Garnish with more fresh berries and that's it! There really is no excuse not to have a filling brekkie. Sort your s**t out, lads.

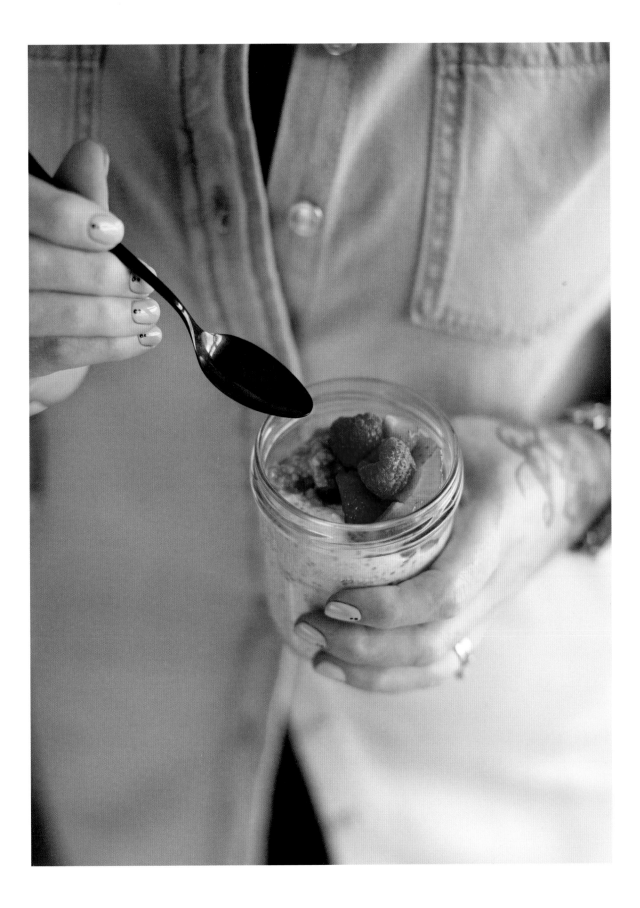

The Perfect
FRIED EGG

So how do you like your eggs in the morning? Cooked ... and cooked properly! I can't be dealing with a raw yolk or that ooey-gooey stuff, it has to be cooked properly on top and there are no eggceptions (I'm sorry).

My mam used to always make our fried eggs this way and it's something I've always done myself; I may not have the aul aluminium lid she used to use but they taste just as good.

SERVES 1

1 egg
1 pan
1 lid

1 If you have a good non-stick pan, no oil is needed for this. I use a small pan (the size of a cracked egg) and it is super handy to keep the shape.

2 Heat your pan on high and crack in the egg. Add a drop of water to the pan, reduce the heat and cover with a lid. The steam from the water will cook the top of the egg evenly so there is no need to flip or pop it under the grill or faff around with it.

3 Cooking time will just depend on how you like your yolk, so keep an eye on it and remove from the heat when it looks just right.

4 You are guaranteed the perfect fried egg every time.

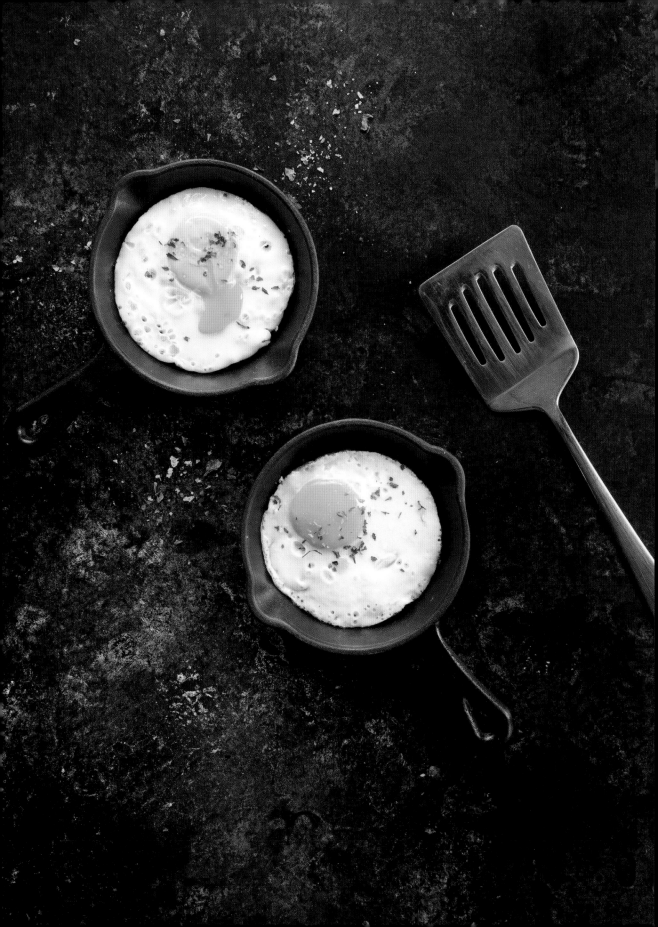

Breakfast BET–

BACON, EGG AND TOMATO TACO

Let face it, tacos are life, so why should they only be for dinner? Let's make them an option for any time of the day. Let me introduce you to the breakfast taco – yes, a taco for breakfast! This will kick-start your day and keep you flying till your next masso meal.

SERVES 2

Low-calorie spray oil

6 cherry tomatoes, chopped

1 tbsp Parmesan cheese, grated

2–3 smoked bacon medallions or American-style bacon

3 eggs, whisked

30ml milk

1 tsp butter

Salt and pepper to taste

2 mini wraps

Hot sauce (optional)

30g Cheddar cheese, grated

1 scallion, sliced (optional)

1 Whack your pan on a high heat and fry the cherry tomatoes with a spray of oil until they start to brown and char, then sprinkle with the Parmesan cheese for a little added flavour – I know, outrageous.

2 Remove from the pan and set to one side, then cook the bacon until nice and crispy. In a different pan, scramble your eggs. Pour them in with the milk and butter, and stir continuously with a spatula. Remove from the heat for a few seconds, stirring, then pop back on the hob and repeat, making sure your eggs don't stick to the bottom of the pan. When your eggs are beginning to scramble, throw in your seasoning, then remove from the heat when they are nice and creamy – don't let them get leathery!

3 Next, we are going to transform a plain Jane wrap into a zingy little ridey wrap bursting with flavour. Pour the hot sauce out on a flat plate and dip the wrap into it on both sides.

4 Heat a clean, non-stick pan on a medium heat and pop the wrap on it for 1–2 minutes, flip and sprinkle one half with half the Cheddar, then half of the scrambled egg, bacon and tomatoes. If using scallions, sprinkle some over too. Fold over to make a taco shape, and keep it on the heat until the cheese is gooey and melty. Repeat with the next wrap and enjoy it all by yourself or with your fella/girl if you are willing to share!

♥

Breakfast

OATIES

Breakfast is my nemesis, and some mornings I don't feel like I can face it but I know I need to get it into me! These fluffy, sweet and filling oaties are handy as you can make them in advance, then they're ready to enjoy with a cuppa in the morning. This recipe serves two and will give you four oaties, two for today and two for tomorrow – handy, dandy! I use a Yorkshire pudding tray to cook mine in but you can make smaller ones with a muffin tray – whatever you have to hand is fine.

SERVES 2

80g porridge oats

2 eggs

70ml skimmed milk

1 tsp baking powder

1 tbsp sweetener

1 tsp vanilla extract

Low-calorie spray oil

4 Biscoff biscuits

1 Preheat your oven to 200°C.

2 Put all the ingredients, except the spray oil and biscuits, into a blender and give it a good blast until you have a nice smooth batter.

3 Grab your pudding or muffin tray and spray a little oil into the four sections you'll be using, just to prevent any sticking. Pour the batter carefully into the cups and lash into the oven for 7 minutes until they start to puff up and rise.

4 At this stage, remove the tin, pop a Biscoff on top of each cup and pop back in the oven for 8 minutes. When they are ready, they should be golden and brown and have a firm texture. Stick on the kettle, make a nice hot cuppa and enjoy!

Cauliflower

POTATO CAKES

Potato cakes are a deadly alternative to chips or just plain aul mash. Served with your favourite meat or just as a snack by themselves with a dip, these will go down a treat. They can be prepared in advance and then heated up, so it's a fuss-free way to get that sneaky veg into the kids.

SERVES 4

300g potatoes, peeled and chopped

150g frozen cauliflower

½ a small onion, finely diced

Low-calorie spray oil

40g Cheddar cheese, freshly grated

Salt to taste

For the coating:

40g instant mash (dry) or panko breadcrumbs

1 tsp turmeric

¼ tsp white pepper

Salt to taste

1 tbsp Grana Padano cheese, grated

Low-calorie spray oil

1 If not using an airfryer, preheat the oven to 200°C.

2 Boil the potatoes in a pot of boiling water until mashable (15–20 minutes). In another pot, cook the cauliflower for the length of time it says on the packet.

3 Drain and mash the spuds then add in the drained, cooked cauliflower and give another mash together.

4 Fry off the onion in a pan with a spray of oil until translucent and add this to the potato and cauliflower mash, then sprinkle in the cheese.

5 Let the mixture cool so you don't burn your hands, then shape into patties. Put on a plate and pop into the fridge for a few hours to stiffen them up and make them easier to coat,

6 To make the coating, mix the instant mash or panko in a bowl with the turmeric, white pepper, salt and cheese; the turmeric will give your cakes a nice yellow colour.

7 Coat the patties in the mash/panko mix.

8 Spray a baking sheet with some low-calorie spray oil, lay out your patties on it, and cook in the preheated oven for 20 minutes, turning halfway through. You can also pop them in the airfryer for 15 minutes until golden and crisp.

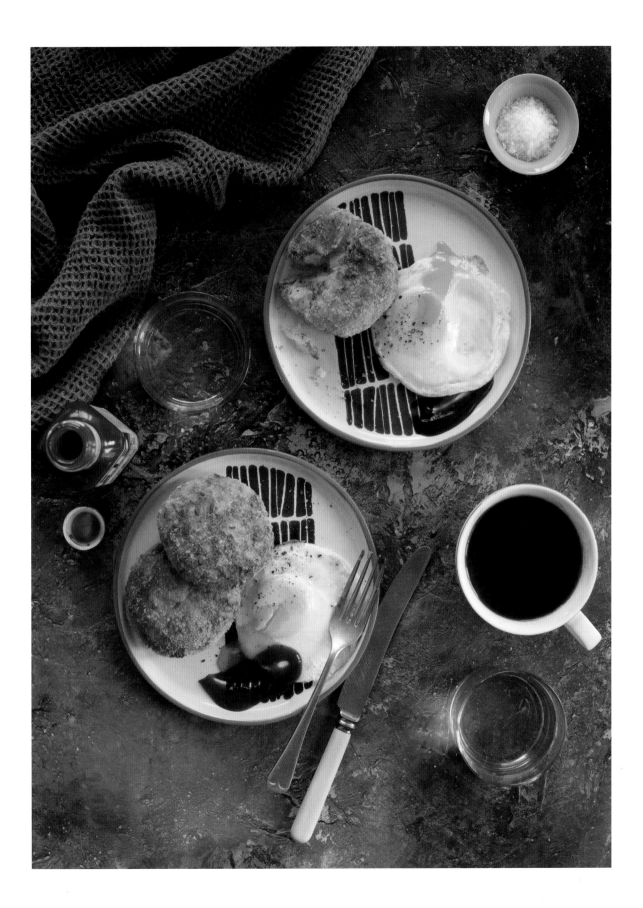

Biscoff

SANDCASTLE

Breakfast, lunch or dessert, you can be guaranteed this will knock the block off any sweet cravings you might have. It feels very, very bold, but when you break it all down it's really not!

SERVES 1

40g porridge oats

1 egg

½ tsp baking powder

50ml skimmed milk

3–4 drops vanilla extract

1 tbsp sweetener

10g Biscoff spread

1 Biscoff biscuit, crumbled

1 Put the oats in a medium-sized microwave-safe mug. Add the rest of the ingredients (apart from the Biscoff spread and biscuit) and give it a good stir, making sure the egg is properly mixed in.

2 Pop the mug in the microwave on a high setting for 3 minutes. The mixture should rise up nice and high and have a spongey texture to touch; if it is still a bit wet, pop it back in for another 30 seconds.

3 Tip out onto a plate.

4 Melt the Biscoff spread in the microwave for 10–15 seconds and drizzle it over the top, then crumble up the biscuit (it looks like sand, hence the 'sand castle') and sprinkle it over the top. Get the biggest spoon you can find and lash it into ya!

Frozen Yoghurt-Dipped
BANANAS

This is such a lovely and healthy treat for the kids (and let's face it, us adults too). You can dip them in your favourite-flavour yoghurt and top with sprinkles or even melted chocolate for an extra treat. These are best prepared the night before, but be sure you make more than enough because everyone will definitely want seconds!

SERVES 8

4 large bananas

1 tub of fat-free Greek yoghurt (I use vanilla)

Lollipop sticks

For the toppings:

Hundreds and thousands

Milk chocolate (melted)

Chopped hazelnuts

1 Peel and cut the bananas into horizontal halves. Get a lollipop stick and push into each half to make them easy to hold.

2 Dip each banana in the yoghurt, covering as much of the banana as you like.

3 Lay out on a flat tray lined with greaseproof paper (ensuring the tray will fit in the freezer) and get your toppings sorted: sprinkle some with hundreds and thousands, drizzle melted chocolate over and sprinkle with some chopped hazelnuts.

4 Pop into the freezer overnight, to be devoured the next morning.

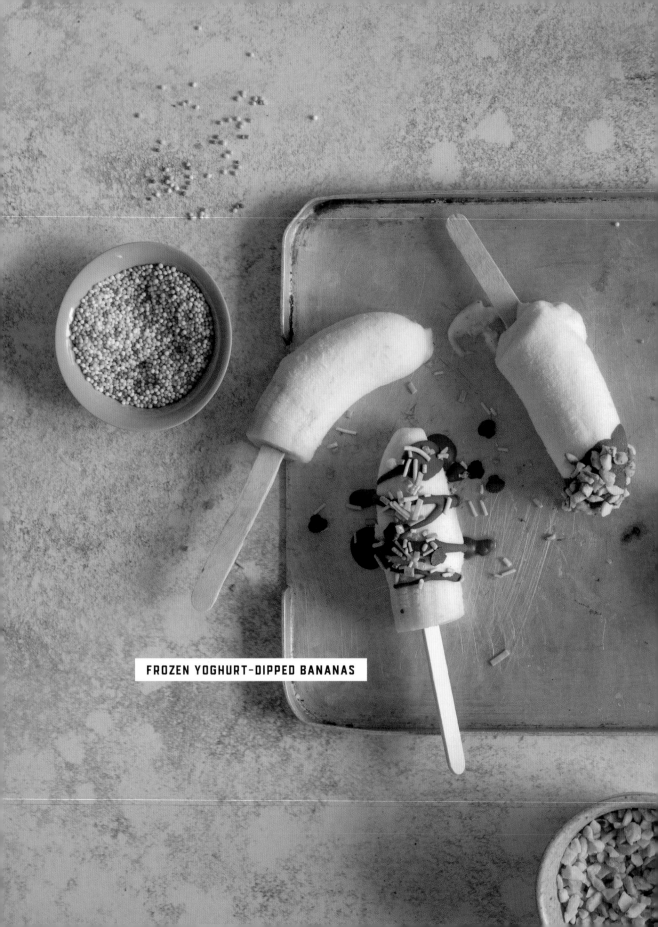

FROZEN YOGHURT-DIPPED BANANAS

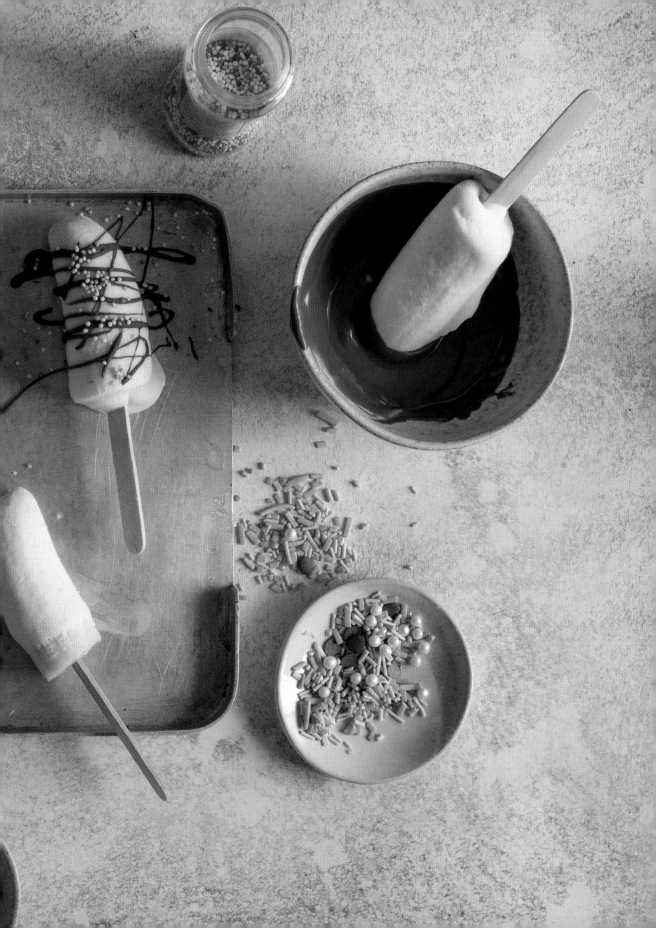

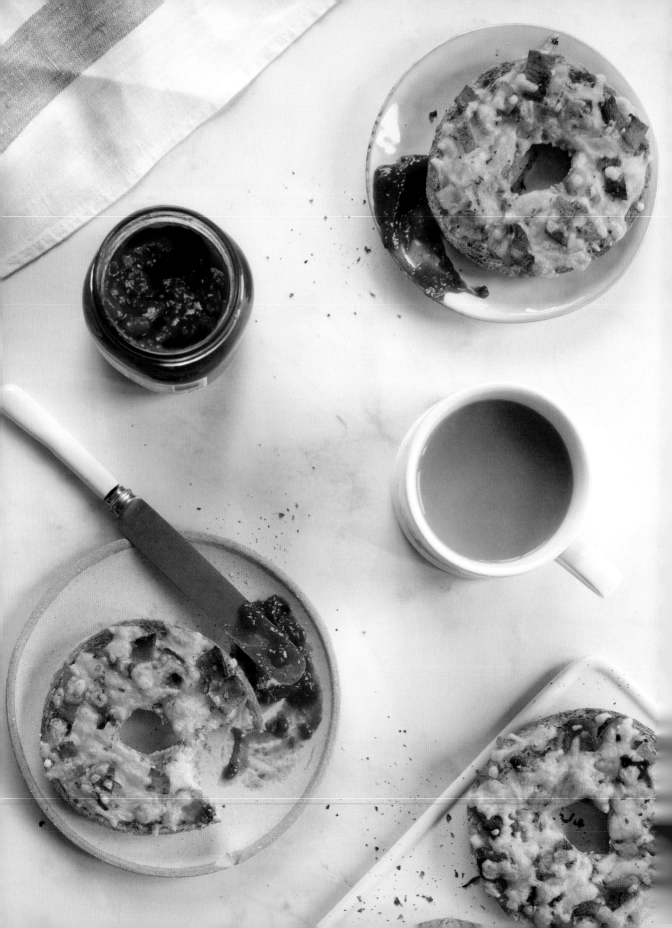

↓

Cheesy Bacon
BREAKFAST BAGELS

If you are stuck for an idea for breakfast, look no further ... I got ya covered! This dish may be very simple and straightforward to prepare, but it's simply delicious! You can grill it or airfry it and it will be ready in under 10 minutes.

SERVES 1

2 bacon medallions

1 wholemeal bagel

30g Cheddar cheese, grated

Tomato relish, to serve

1 Start by grilling or airfrying the bacon medallions, then when cooked, chop them up.

2 Slice the bagel in half and lay out, inside facing up. Sprinkle the Cheddar cheese and the chopped bacon over both halves.

3 Pop under the grill or into the airfryer for 5–6 minutes or until the cheese is melted and golden.

4 Serve with some tomato relish.

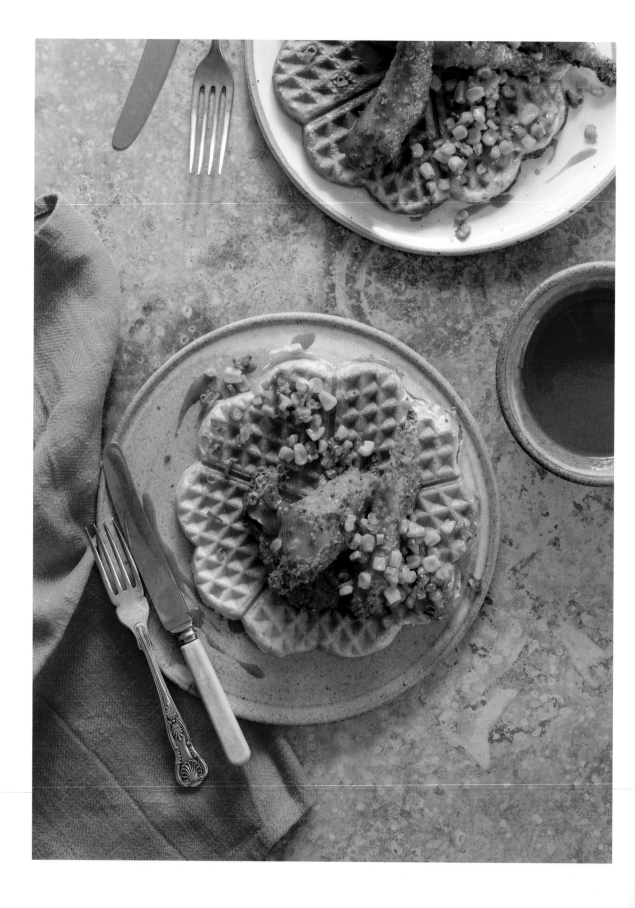

Buffalo Chicken and Waffles with
ROASTED SWEETCORN

A midweek treat or weekend fakeaway, this deadly recipe will be loved by everyone, and is super easy to recreate! You'll need a waffle maker to make it.

SERVES 4

For the buffalo chicken:

30g panko breadcrumbs

1 tsp garlic granules

Salt and black pepper to taste or 1 tbsp lemon pepper

Low-calorie spray oil

3–4 chicken breasts, sliced into strips

1 small tin of sweetcorn, drained

200ml buffalo hot sauce

1 tbsp sweetener

1 tsp vinegar

1 tsp butter

For the waffle batter:

120g plain flour

237ml milk

1 tbsp sweetener

½ tbsp baking powder

1 egg

Low-calorie spray oil

To serve:

Roasted sweetcorn

A few scallions, thinly sliced

1 Preheat the oven to 220°C.

2 In a bowl, mix the panko with the seasoning. Spray the chicken pieces with some oil and massage it in, then coat with the seasoned panko. Lay out on a baking sheet lined with greaseproof paper and pop in the preheated oven for 20–25 minutes, turning halfway through. Five minutes before it's cooked, spread your sweetcorn out on a small baking tray and pop in the oven until golden.

3 When the chicken is nearly ready, heat the hot sauce in a high-sided pan with the sweetener, vinegar and butter. When the chicken is cooked, toss it into the sauce until fully coated. Set aside while you prepare the waffles.

4 Pop the flour, milk, sweetener, baking powder and egg into a blender and blitz until smooth.

5 Preheat your waffle maker and give it a light spray with the oil. Pour the batter into the waffle maker, being careful not to overfill it.

6 Cook for 4–5 minutes until golden and brown.

7 Once the chicken is ready, serve on top of the hot waffles and sprinkle over the roasted sweetcorn and the scallions.

Chicken Fajita
PROTEIN SALAD BOWL

When I think of protein bowls I think of power and strength, so that's exactly what should be packed into these. We don't want limp lettuce and a few measly bits of veg scattered around. We want crunch and bite with lots of fresh, crisp veg. Choosing what to use is totally to your own taste but you want to make sure it's full of greens, raw veggies, beans if possible and a healthy grain; I am using brown rice.

SERVES 2

150g pre-cooked roast chicken pieces

½ tsp smoked paprika

½ tsp garlic granules

½ tsp chilli powder

Salt and pepper to taste

250g pre-cooked wholegrain rice

1 red onion, sliced

1 red pepper, deseeded and sliced

1 green pepper, deseeded and sliced

A handful of cherry tomatoes, halved

½ a lettuce, leaves separated

1 avocado, sliced

1 small tin of sweetcorn, drained

Fresh coriander (if it's your thing)

1 lime for juice and garnish

2 tbsp sour cream

1 Toss the chicken in a warm pan with the spices and salt and pepper to taste until coated and warmed through. If you prefer, you can omit the spices and simply warm the chicken.
2 Heat the rice as per the packet instructions. You can fry off the onion, peppers and tomatoes if you prefer less bite.
3 Next all you need to do is get your assembly skills at the ready and build your bowl. Into each bowl, I pop the lettuce first then the rice (half the pack) and tuck it into one side, then I load in all my veggies and chicken. I finish with some fresh coriander, a squeeze of lime over the top and a wedge to garnish, and a dollop of cool sour cream. Masso.

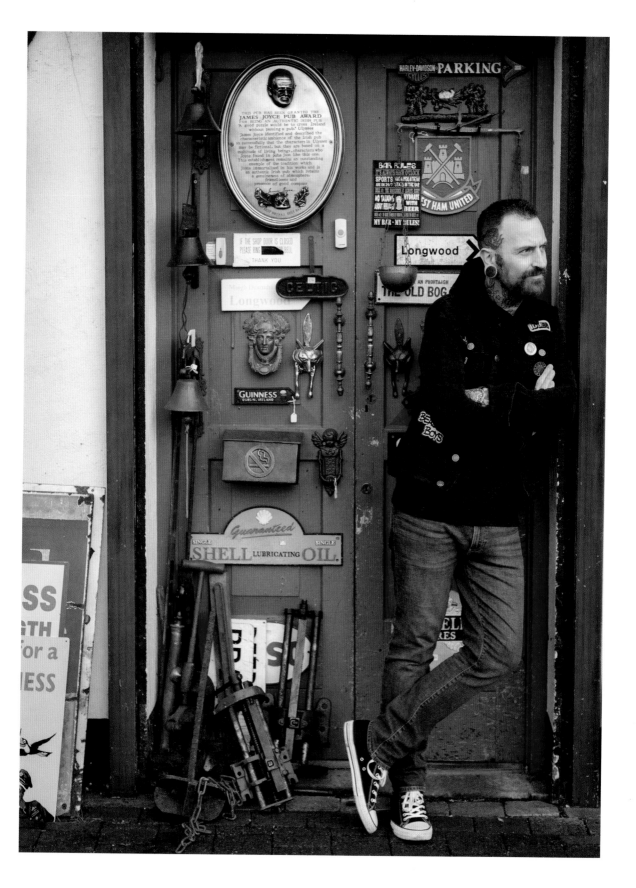

Aubergine
HUMMUS

This smoky little beauty is a fabulous starter or lunch served with crisped-up wholemeal pitta to dip and devour! I've combined two of my loves, roasted aubergines and roasted garlic, to make this incredible hummus.

SERVES LOADS

1 aubergine, cut in half (from the stalk down)

2 garlic cloves, peeled

Low-calorie spray oil

1 x 400g tin of chickpeas, drained

1 tsp sesame oil (optional)

Juice of ½ a lemon

Salt to taste

To garnish:

Smoked paprika

Fresh parsley

1 Preheat the oven to 200°C.

2 Pop the aubergine and garlic on a baking tray with a little spray oil and cook for 35–40 minutes until the aubergine is soft and scoopable, and the garlic has browned.

3 Remove from the oven, let cool a little, then scoop out the flesh into a blender, add the garlic and the rest of the ingredients and blend until smooth. You can add some water little by little if it is too thick, until you get your desired consistency.

4 Serve in a bowl and garnish with a shake of smoked paprika and some parsley scattered over. Perfect as a dip with some homemade flatbread (see page 179).

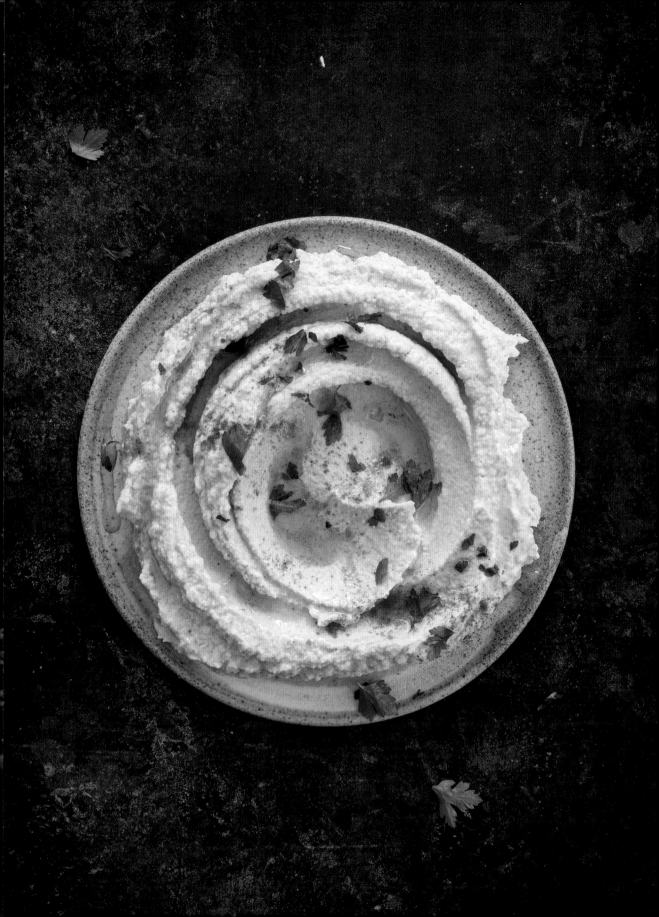

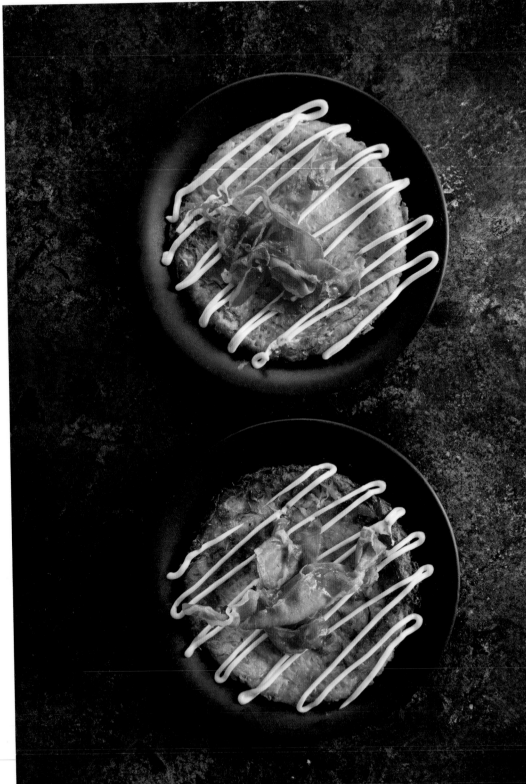

OKONOMIYAKI

O-ko-no-me what now? Well it's essentially a pancake – a savoury one. This Japanese dish is absolutely packed with flavour. The name comes from the Japanese word 'okonomi' which means how/what you like and the word 'yaki' which means cooked. There are loads of different variations of okonomiyaki that I've seen and this is my particular take on it. It's perfect for any meal of the day but for me this one is a great weekend brunch treat.

SERVES 2

200ml vegetable stock

2 eggs

2 tbsp soy sauce

100g plain flour

2 scallions, finely sliced

1 carrot, sliced into long, thin strips

½ a savoy cabbage, sliced into long, thin strips

1 fresh red chilli, deseeded and chopped

1 tsp Japanese 7 spice

Low-calorie spray oil

4 slices of prosciutto, sliced into thin strips

1 Get your stock, eggs and soy sauce into a mixing bowl and whisk everything up. Start to gradually add your flour and keep on whisking until you have a nice smooth mixture with no lumps.

2 Throw all your prepared veg into the bowl along with the Japanese 7 spice and mix everything together.

3 Grab your frying pan, throw in a little oil, pop on a medium heat and add half your mixture to the pan. Think of it like you're making a pancake, so you want it to have that circular shape. Give it about 4–5 minutes then flip over (use a fish slice to help), then give another 4–5 minutes to cook the other side. You can pop on a lid on the pan while cooking as this help it to cook fully throughout.

4 Lastly, spread your prosciutto evenly across the top of your cooked mix and then pop under the grill for 1–2 minutes just to crisp up. Repeat for the second 'pancake'.

5 Serve and enjoy. Goes great with some Japanese mayo or sweet chilli sauce.

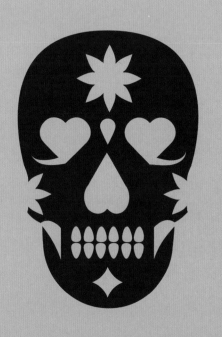

MAMBO
SAMBO

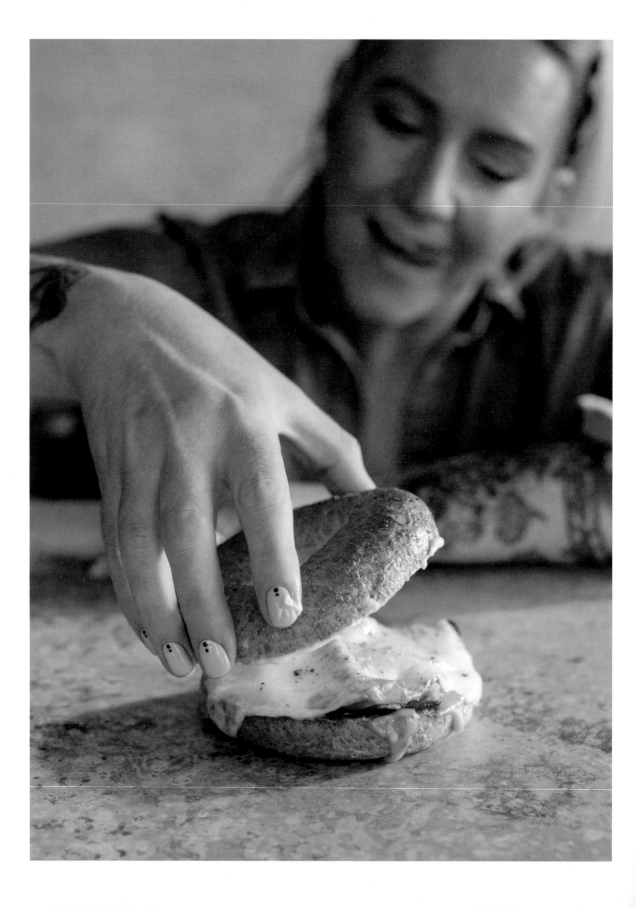

Cubano

BAGEL

One sandwich I always loved was the Cubano. A bar that I used to frequent served a great one and it went down a treat with a cold beer. Here's an easier and healthier take on this classic sambo.

SERVES I

1 wholemeal bagel, sliced in half

1 tbsp yellow mustard

1 tbsp lighter than light mayo

2 slices of fresh carved ham or deli ham

1 gherkin, sliced lengthways

10g mozzarella cheese, grated

10g Cheddar cheese, grated

Salt and pepper to taste

1 First off give your bagel halves around 60 seconds in the toaster to get them warmed up. Spread the yellow mustard over the bottom half, and the mayo over the top half. Now start to build your bagel: get your ham down over the mustardy half, followed by your gherkin slices and both cheeses.

2 Stick this half under a grill for a minute or so, just to get the cheese starting to melt. Remove, sprinkle over a little salt and pepper, then pop the top half of the bagel on.

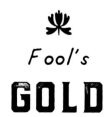

Fool's
GOLD

What is fool's gold, you may ask. Well, c'mere and let me tell you the legend of the fool's gold sandwich. This was originally made by a restaurant in Denver, Colorado and gained fame as it was one of Elvis Presley's favourite things to eat. Back then, the sandwich was made with a hollowed-out loaf of French white bread filled with one jar of peanut butter (yup, a full jar), one jar of grape jam and then a pound of bacon – everything a growing person needs, right?

So here's our toned-down, healthier version. It's still a treat to have but nowhere near as calorific as the original one. This is a firm fave with our kids.

SERVES 2

4 bacon medallions
Low-calorie spray oil
4 slices of wholemeal bread
Light butter
4 tbsp peanut butter
4 tbsp sugar-free strawberry jam

Elvis music playing in the background (optional)

1 Cut your bacon into strips and cook in a non-stick pan with a spray of oil until crispy.
2 Next up, grab your four slices of bread and give each slice a light coating of butter on one side. Flip the slices over and cover two with the jam and the other two with the peanut butter (remember we're making two sambos here).
3 Grab your bacon and arrange evenly on top of the peanut butter. Close off the sandwiches (jammy sides over the bacon), pop a pan on a medium heat and whack in a little spray oil. Toast each side of the sandwiches for around two minutes – you just want to get them a little bit crisped up and warm.
4 Serve and enjoy – you'll be singing 'Blue Suede Shoes' around the kitchen for the rest of the day.

Lime

CHICKEN WRAP

My love of wraps continues with this Mexican-inspired little beauty. Makes a great lunch or epic dinner served with some Perfect Chips (see page 6).

If making this for lunch what I would do is get the chicken boiled the night before, let it cool and pop it in the fridge. That way it'll only take about five minutes to get this wrap made up.

SERVES 1

1 chicken fillet

3 tbsp salsa

Juice of 1 lime

1 tsp chilli flakes

½ tsp garlic granules

½ tsp smoked paprika

1 wholemeal wrap

6 jalapeño slices (from a jar)

10g mozzarella cheese, grated

10g Cheddar cheese, grated

1 tbsp sour cream

¼ head of lettuce, shredded

1 Put your chicken fillet in a pot of boiling water and leave to simmer for 35–40 minutes. When cooked, drain off any excess water and, using two forks, shred it up.

2 Get a saucepan and throw in your chicken, salsa, lime juice, chilli flakes, garlic granules and paprika. Place on a low to medium heat and stir everything together, until it's nice and warmed up.

3 Lay out your wrap and spoon the chicken and sauce in a straight line along the inside. Scatter over the jalapeños and both cheeses and pop under the grill for a minute or two to allow the cheese to melt.

4 Take out from under the grill, add the sour cream and lettuce, wrap up, cut in half and enjoy.

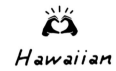

Hawaiian
GAMMON SANDWICH

Aloha, here's a sandwich that packs a tropical punch and will have you doing the hula around the kitchen. Well, maybe not, but it's a great handy lunch and packed with flavour.

SERVES 1

1 gammon steak

2 slices of fresh pineapple

2 slices of wholemeal bread

1 tbsp lighter than light mayo

2 slices of light Cheddar cheese

1 Cook your gammon steak on the pan and just as it's finished throw on your pineapple slices too. You just want to give them a little blast on each side to warm them up and char them slightly.

2 Grab your bread and spread your mayo on one slice. Pile on your gammon, cheese slices and pineapple and top with the other slice.

3 Serve and enjoy.

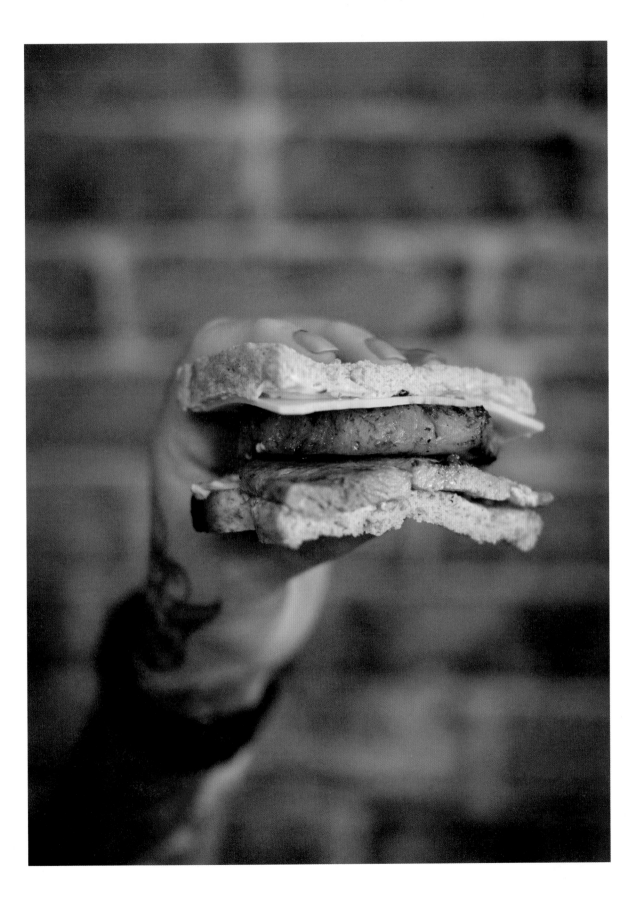

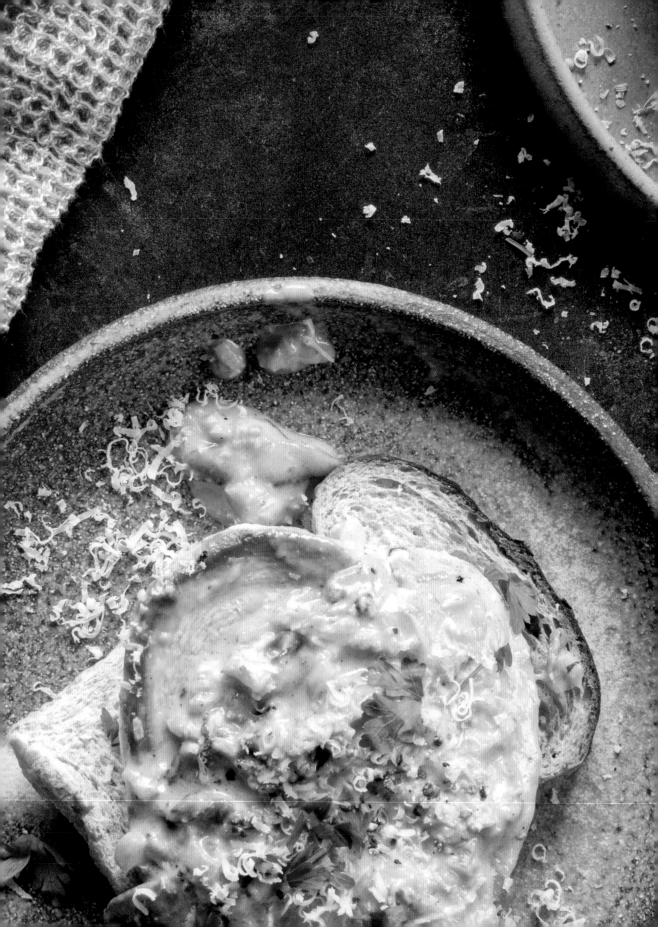

Italian

CHICKEN SAMBO

This Italian-inspired chicken fillet sandwich is packed full of flavour. We had something similar while staying in Rome and ever since I wanted to do my own take on it. It's juicy, creamy and literally dripping with flavour. Great for lunch or just as good as a dinner served alongside some homemade fries (see Perfect Chips, page 6).

SERVES 2

2 chicken fillets

Low-calorie spray oil

2 tbsp oil (I use rapeseed)

3 garlic cloves, finely sliced

8–10 mushrooms, sliced

1/2 fresh red chilli, deseeded and finely sliced (optional)

1/2 fresh green chilli, deseeded and finely sliced (optional)

1 onion, halved and sliced

300ml chicken stock

125ml light cream

60–100g Parmesan cheese, grated

Cornflour (optional)

Salt and pepper to taste

4 slices of wholemeal bread

1 Get your chicken fillets and butterfly them (see page 36 for instructions), give a light spray with oil and get them cooking on a pan on a medium heat for around 8 minutes per side. Set aside while you get on with the rest of the sandwich filling.

2 To cook the veg, get another pan on a medium heat and give a few sprays of oil. As the pan heats, throw in your garlic and give it a minute to infuse with the oil, then add the mushrooms and give them around 2 minutes to cook with the garlic and oil. Finally add in the chilli (if using) and onion.

3 Let the veg cook for a few minutes, stirring as you go – you want to see your onions going translucent. When this happens add your stock, cream and Parmesan, keeping the pan on a medium heat for a further 4–5 minutes. If your sauce seems watery, add a little cornflour (first mixed to a paste with some water in a cup) to thicken up. You want a nice creamy consistency. Season with salt and pepper.

4 When your sauce is ready, transfer it into a mixing bowl. One by one, add the cooked chicken pieces, making sure you coat them evenly in the mixture.

5 Get your bread and lightly toast it then put each saucy chicken fillet on a slice, adding excess sauce on top – yup, this is gonna be messy but it will be so worth it.

6 Top with the other slice of bread and cut in half, then repeat to make the second sandwich. Serve and enjoy.

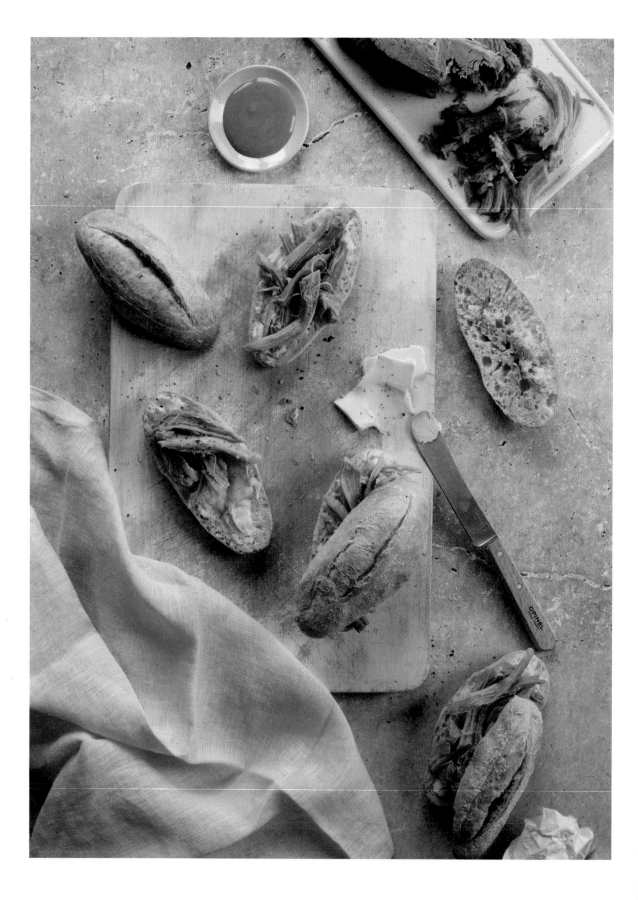

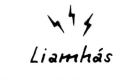

Liamhás
AGUS IM

One of our most travelled to – and favourite – cities over the years is Paris. It's a city filled with romance, beautiful architecture, endless sights and some amazing food. We've been lucky to eat in some fab restaurants in Paris but one of our favourite eats from this city is the famous jambon-beurre, which is simply ham and butter served on a fresh baguette. So simple, but when made right it's a delight to eat and every time I make one it brings me right back to Paris. We've put our take on the popular French classic so without further ado, we present the 'Liamhás agus Im' (Irish for 'ham and butter').

SERVES 2

Unsmoked ham fillet (between 500 and 700g)

1 x 330ml can of Coke Zero

2 x fresh (warm) demi baguettes (or 1 full baguette, halved)

Real butter

Dijon mustard (optional)

1 I usually prepare my ham the night before. I pop the fillet into the slow cooker, add the can of Coke and leave it on low to cook overnight (roughly 8 hours); Coke gives the fillet an extra sweetness and flavour kick. If you don't have a slow cooker, you can simply boil it on the hob according to instructions. The great thing about using a fillet is that you'll have plenty left over – pop it in the fridge and make more sandwiches during the week or give the kids some epic ham sambos for school.

2 To make your roll, get your demi baguettes (or halved baguette) and slice lengthways down the middle. I always pop it under the grill for a minute or two just to get it warm and a little crisped up.

3 Traditionally this would be served with loads of butter lashed on but obviously use as much or as little as you like, I lightly coat one side of the inside with butter, then I add 3–4 nice thick slices of ham. That's it, there you have it.

4 For some additional flavour add a little Dijon mustard.

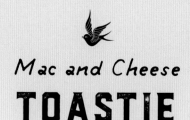

Mac and Cheese
TOASTIE

Here's a toastie that'll fill you up: creamy, yummy mac and cheese lashed into a grilled sambo.

SERVES 2

100-120g macaroni

3 light cheese single slices, torn

30g Cheddar cheese, grated

50ml water

Light butter

4 slices of wholemeal bread

Salt and pepper to taste

Low-calorie spray oil

1 Put your pasta in a saucepan with water and a pinch of salt and cook for the amount of time it says on the packet.

2 While the pasta is cooking, get another medium-sized saucepan and pop your cheese singles and Cheddar in with the water. Cook on a low to medium heat and stir until it's all melted together and smooth.

3 Once your cheese sauce is ready, put to the side and get your pasta organised. Fully drain and shake off any excess water, then drop it into the pot with the cheese sauce and mix together, coating everything evenly.

4 Lightly butter the 4 slices of bread on one side, scoop half the mix onto one slice (the unbuttered side). Season with a little salt and pepper and put the top slice on (buttered side up). Repeat with the other two slices.

5 Have a pan on a medium heat and add a spray of oil. Let it heat up and add the sandwiches, then let them cook for a couple of minutes on each side until they are golden brown. Enjoy! If you fancy it, you can add some cooked, chopped bacon to the mac and cheese at the mixing stage for extra flavour.

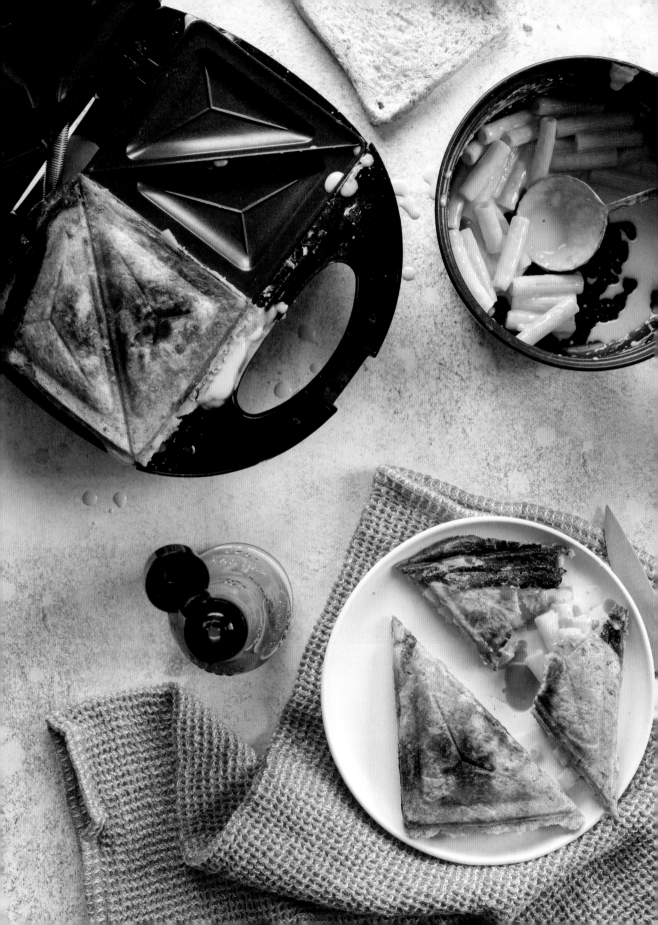

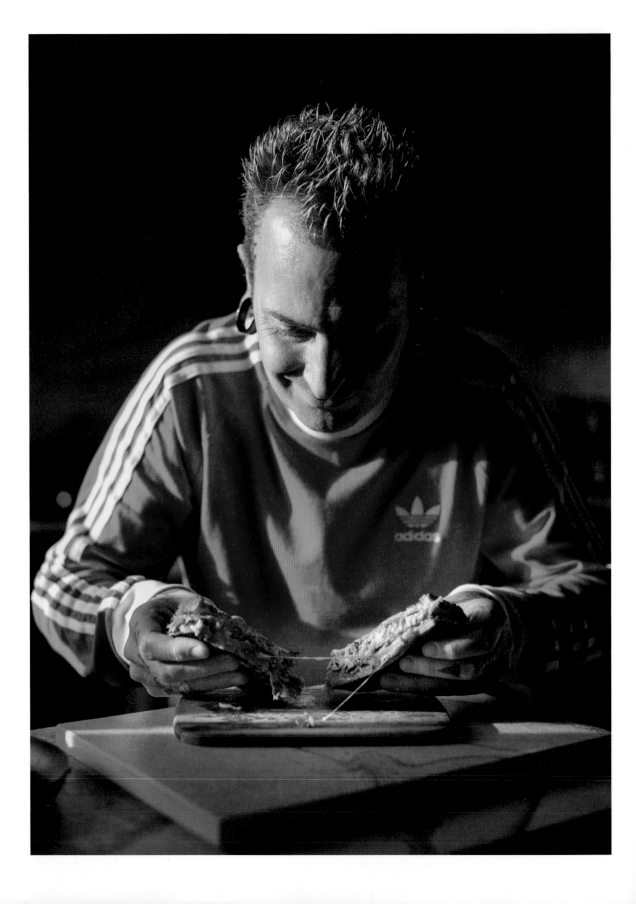

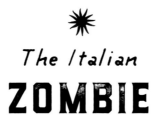

The Italian
ZOMBIE

My love of zombie movies and grilled cheese sambos come head to head here with the whopper Italian zombie. This will fill the hungriest of tummies and set your taste buds hopping, great for lunch or brunch.

SERVES 1

2 slices of wholemeal bread

Light butter

2 tbsp zombie slaw (see page 73)

2 slices of prosciutto

¼ onion, diced

1 gherkin, sliced into circles

15g mozzarella cheese, grated

15g Cheddar cheese, grated

3–4 slices of roasted red peppers (from a jar)

Low-calorie spray oil

1 Get your bread and lightly butter each slice on one side. Add your slaw, prosciutto, onion, gherkin, both cheeses and peppers and pop the top slice on (keeping the buttered sides on the outside).

2 Get your pan onto a medium heat and give it a spray of oil. Pop your sambo in and cook for around 2–3 minutes on each side until it goes a nice golden colour.

3 Serve and enjoy.

Maple Bacon and Egg
GRILLED CHEESE

Here's another scrumptious grilled cheese recipe. The egg is the secret weapon here, adding a lovely gooey texture to this sweet and savoury sandwich. Pure delight with every bite.

SERVES 1

3 bacon medallions

Low-calorie spray oil

1 tbsp maple syrup

1 egg

2 slices of wholemeal bread

Light butter

15g mozzarella cheese, grated

15g Cheddar cheese, grated

1 Slice your bacon into strips, get a pan on a medium heat and give it a couple of sprays of oil. Lash on your bacon and cook through, drizzling over the maple syrup as it cooks.

2 While your bacon is cooking get another pan and get your fried egg on too – you want it nice and runny on the inside (see page 96).

3 Get your bread and lightly butter each slice on the outside. Put your bacon, both cheeses and egg inside and pop the top slice on.

4 Get a clean pan onto a medium head and give it a spray of oil. Put this baby in and cook for around 2–3 minutes on each side until it goes a nice golden colour.

5 Serve and enjoy.

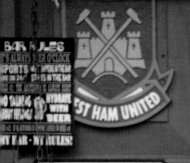

BAR RULES

Longwood

AR AN FHUTAIGH
THE OLD BOG ROAD 2

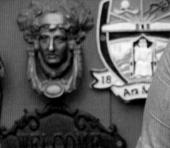

WELCOME

GUINNESS
DUBLIN, IRELAND

GUINNESS
EXTRA STOUT

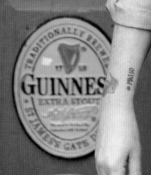

MICHELIN
TYRES

Faux

PULLED PORK

BBQ pulled pork is a thing of beauty and can be used in so many ways – as a burger, as a filling for a jacket potato or piled high on top of fries for a loaded feast! However, making it from scratch can take some time and when time is of the essence but you need pulled pork … we reinvented it and created a little timesaving hack! Okay, okay, I know it's not exactly the same but it does the feckin' trick. Once you know the hack, you can make masso sambos with it, like the one below!

SERVES 2-4

1 packet of sliced ham

2 tbsp BBQ sauce

That's literally it!

For the masso cheese toastie:

Light butter or low-calorie spray oil

2 slices of wholemeal bread

Whatever cheese you fancy, grated

1 Empty the pack of ham onto a chopping board and, using a sharp knife, slice it up as finely as you can.

2 Heat a pan on the hob and throw in the ham. Add the BBQ sauce and mix it through well. Then it's ready!

3 Butter two slices of bread on one side or spray with some oil. Heat a pan and place one slice of the bread in, buttered side down. Add a sprinkle or a handful of cheese, whatever you're into. Add some faux pork and then the other slice of bread on top (buttered side out).

4 Flip after 2–3 minutes and repeat on the other side until the cheese is all melty and delicious.

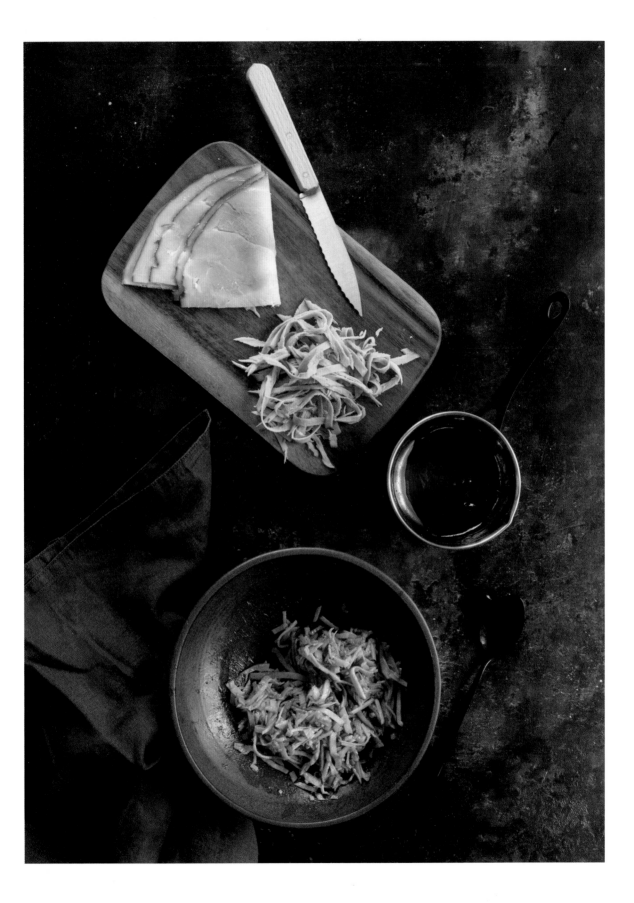

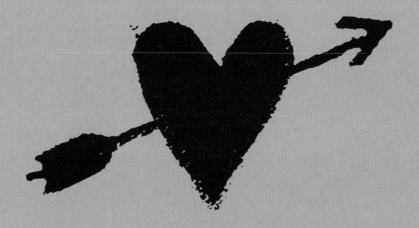

WHAT'S THE SOUP?

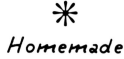

Homemade

VEGETABLE SOUP

This super-basic recipe is wholesome, thick and tasty and perfect to store in the fridge for a few days if you have any leftovers. Like all my soup recipes, you can add in some leftover chicken to bulk it up and give some extra protein and filling power.

SERVES 4-6

Low-calorie spray oil

1 onion, finely diced

2 garlic cloves, minced

3 carrots, chopped

1 head of fresh broccoli, chopped

2 medium-sized potatoes, peeled and cut into cubes

750ml chicken stock

½ tsp dried thyme

Salt and pepper to taste

1 Start by sautéing the onion and garlic in a large pot sprayed with some oil until the onion is translucent.

2 Add in the carrots, broccoli and potatoes and fry off for a few minutes, stirring well.

3 Add in the chicken stock and thyme and season with salt and pepper to taste. Bring to the boil then simmer for 10–12 minutes, until the veg are soft enough to blend.

4 Taste and add more seasoning if needed, then use a hand blender to blend until you have a smooth consistency.

5 Serve in warm bowls with some crusty breast and real butter for a little treat. Yum!

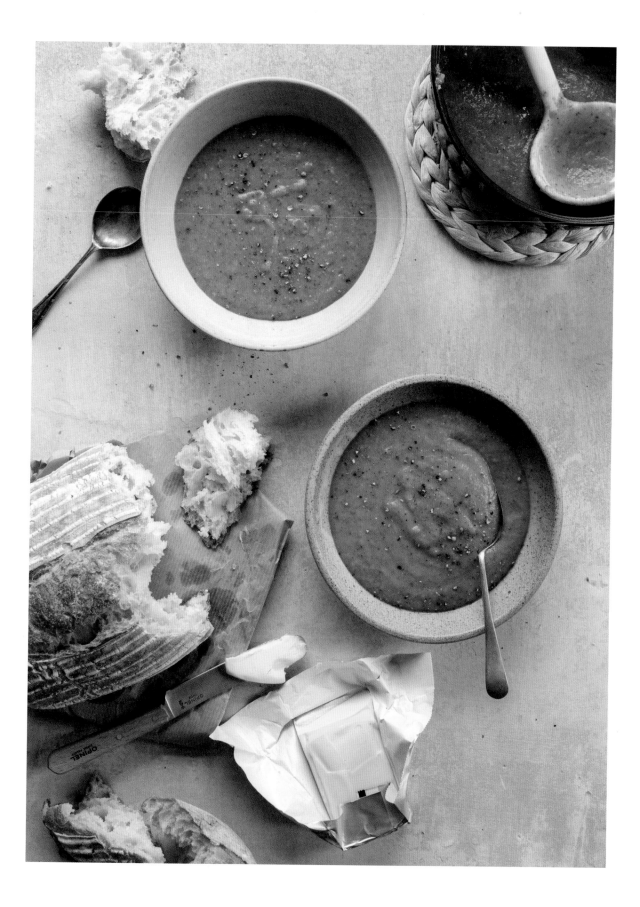

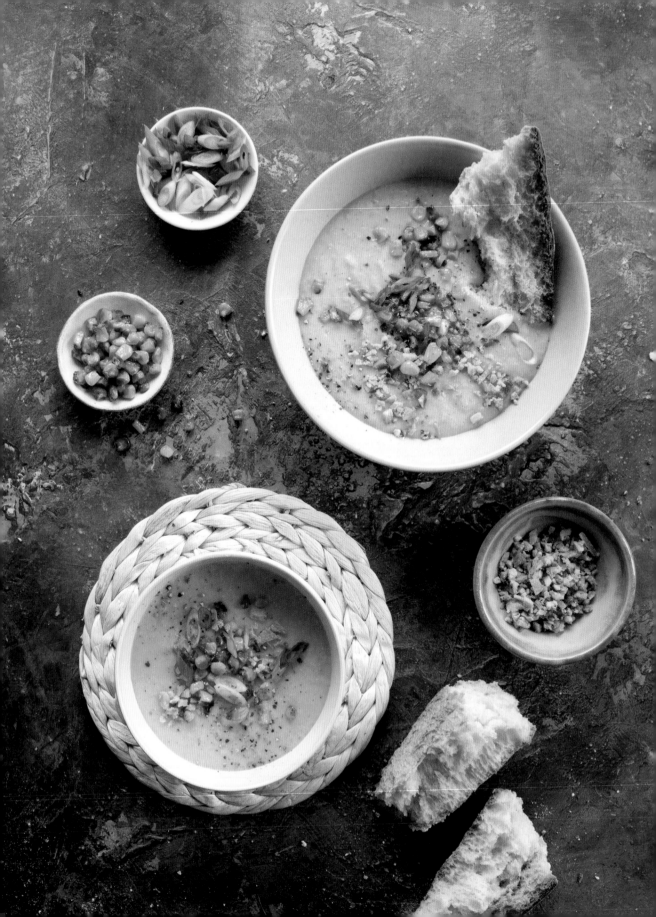

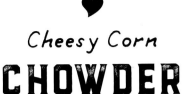

Cheesy Corn
CHOWDER

Thick and creamy sweetcorn soup is absolutely delicious, and garnishing it with smoky bacon crumbs and charred sweetcorn gives it an extra depth of flavour. Expect this to become a weekly winner in your gaff. For extra protein add in some cooked, shredded chicken.

SERVES 4-6

4 smoked bacon medallions or American-style bacon

2 x 340g tins of sweetcorn, drained

Low-calorie spray oil

1 onion, finely diced

2 sticks of celery, diced

1 carrot, diced

1 tbsp flour

1 large potato, peeled and cut into cubes

600ml chicken stock

200ml milk

60g Cheddar cheese, grated

½ tsp smoked paprika

1 tsp garlic powder

½ tsp dried thyme

Salt and pepper to taste

1 Pop your choice of bacon under the grill or in the airfryer at 190°C until crispy and brown, finely chop and set aside.

2 Pop half a tin of sweetcorn in the airfryer at 190°C until golden and crisp or spread out on a baking sheet and put under the grill, turning occasionally so it doesn't burn, until charred and golden. Set aside until the soup is ready.

3 Next sauté the onion, celery and carrot in a large pot with a little spray of oil, stirring until tender. Sprinkle over the flour, which will thicken the soup, and mix.

4 Add in the cubed potato and the remaining sweetcorn, and fry off for 2–3 minutes.

5 Add in the chicken stock, milk, Cheddar, smoked paprika, garlic powder and thyme and season with salt and pepper to taste.

6 Simmer for 10–12 minutes until the cheese has melted in and combined with the stock, and the potatoes are tender enough to blend.

7 Taste and add more seasoning if needed, then use a hand blender to blend until smooth.

8 Serve in warm bowls and sprinkle the bacon crumbs and charred sweetcorn on top.

★ ★ ★

Roasted

CARROT AND GINGER SOUP

Here's a lovely little belly warmer for when the colder evenings start creeping in. It's like a massive hug in a bowl. Perfect to batch cook and keep in the fridge or portion out and freeze for when you need it.

SERVES 6

1 kg carrots, chopped in half, then in half again

Low-calorie spray oil

1 small onion, finely diced

2–3 garlic cloves, minced

1 litre chicken stock

½ tsp ground ginger

¼ tsp chilli flakes

Salt and pepper to taste

½ tsp Aromat seasoning

A knob of butter (optional)

1 Preheat the oven to 220°C.

2 Lay out your carrots on a baking sheet lined with greaseproof paper, spray with a little spray oil and pop in the preheated oven for 40 minutes until soft and beginning to caramelise.

3 Meanwhile, heat a large pot on a medium heat with a spray of oil and add in the onion and garlic. Sweat them off until the onion becomes translucent.

4 When the carrots are ready, add them to the pot along with the stock, ginger, chilli flakes, salt and pepper, Aromat and butter (if you're using it).

5 Give everything a good stir, simmer for 10 minutes then blend with a hand blender until smooth.

6 Serve in a warm bowl with some brown bread – delish!

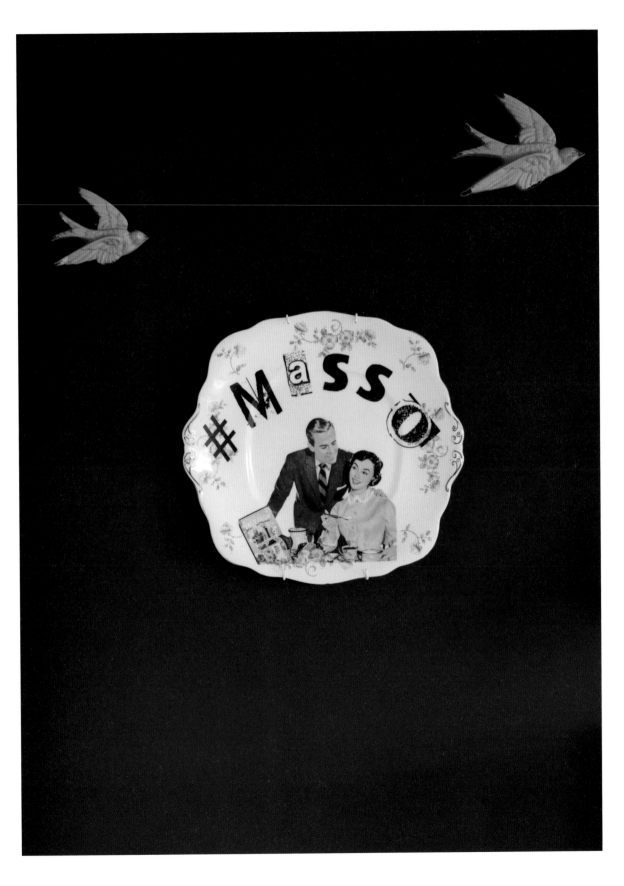

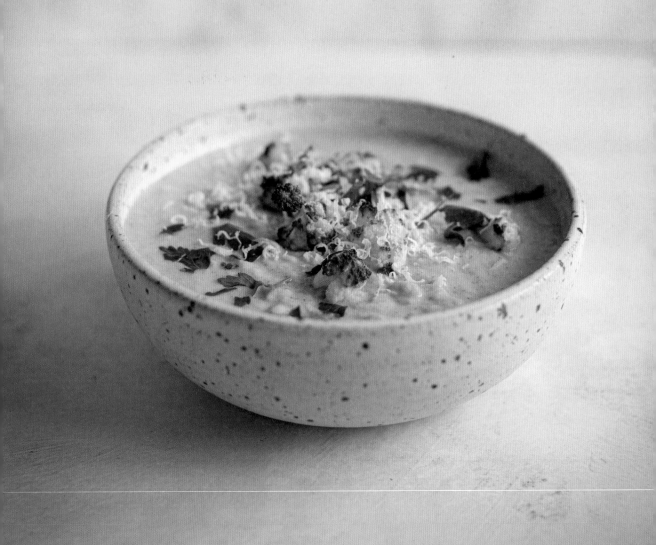

Roasted Cauliflower and Garlic
SOUP

Cauliflower is one of my favourite vegetables, and roasting it gives it such a beautiful, unique flavour. Roasting the garlic, as we do in this recipe, brings everything to a whole new level with its subtle sweetness. This is one page you'll be earmarking for sure.

SERVES 6

2 cauliflower heads, broken up

1 bulb of garlic, top cut off to expose the cloves

Low-calorie spray oil

½ an onion, finely diced

1 litre chicken or veg stock (I used chicken)

100ml light cream

Salt and pepper to taste

To garnish:

Fresh parsley, chopped

Parmesan cheese, grated

1 Preheat the oven to 220°C.

2 Lay out the cauliflower on a baking tray lined with greaseproof paper and pop the garlic on there too, cut side up. Spray it all with some oil and roast in the preheated oven for 40 minutes, until the cauliflower is tender and slightly charred and the garlic is golden and softened.

3 In a large pot sprayed with some oil, fry off the onion until translucent. Throw in the roasted cauliflower and squeeze the garlic out of its skin, being careful not to burn your hands. Pour in the stock, bring to a boil, then cover and simmer for 10–15 minutes.

4 Add the cream and salt and pepper to taste, then blitz until smooth. If it's too thick, add a little water.

5 Serve in warm bowls with a sprinkle of parsley and some Parmesan. Gorgeous!

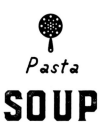

Pasta

SOUP

This one is perfect for those cold, wintry days; comforting and nourishing. There's something about chicken and chorizo; they just go so well together – the flavours set each other off and it's a taste I'll never tire of.

SERVES 2

Low-calorie spray oil

350g chicken mini fillets, diced

2 garlic cloves, minced

4 nests of tagliatelle

200g mushrooms, finely diced

60g chorizo, diced

1 x 400g tin of cream of chicken soup

½ tsp smoked paprika

30g Parmesan cheese, grated

1 Spray a pan with some oil and brown off your chicken with the garlic, throwing a shot of water into the pan while cooking to deglaze and get all the tasty bits off the bottom.

2 When your chicken is cooking get your pasta into a pot of salted boiling water (follow the instructions on the packet).

3 Throw in your shrooms with the chicken and fry off, then lash in your chorizo. Once the chicken and chorizo are cooked, add your tin of soup and cook on a low heat, mixing everything together well, until heated through. Lastly, pop in your paprika and Parmesan. As you cook it will reduce down, so add a little water if needed.

4 Drain off your pasta and add into the pan with your chicken and chorizo and mix everything together.

5 Serve up and enjoy.

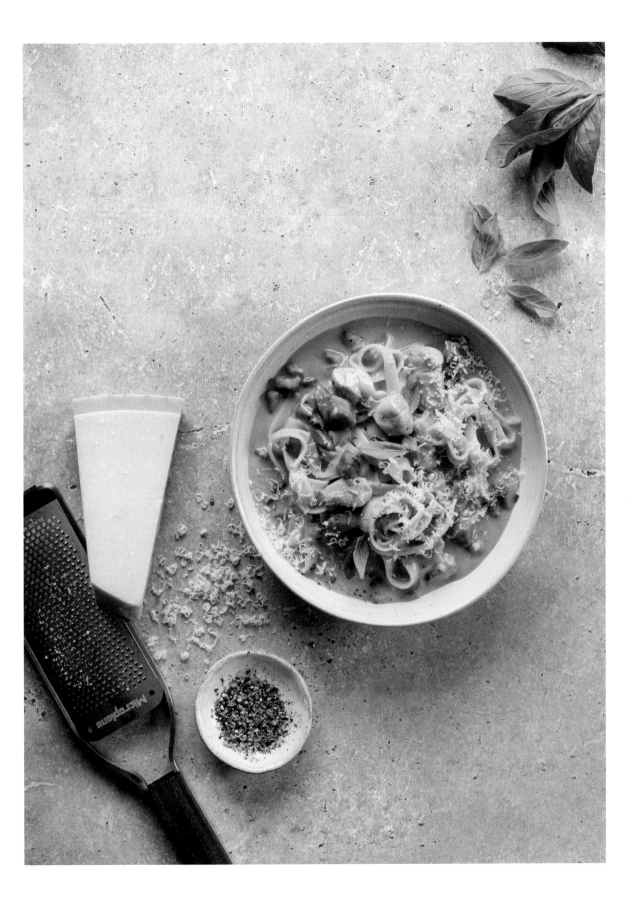

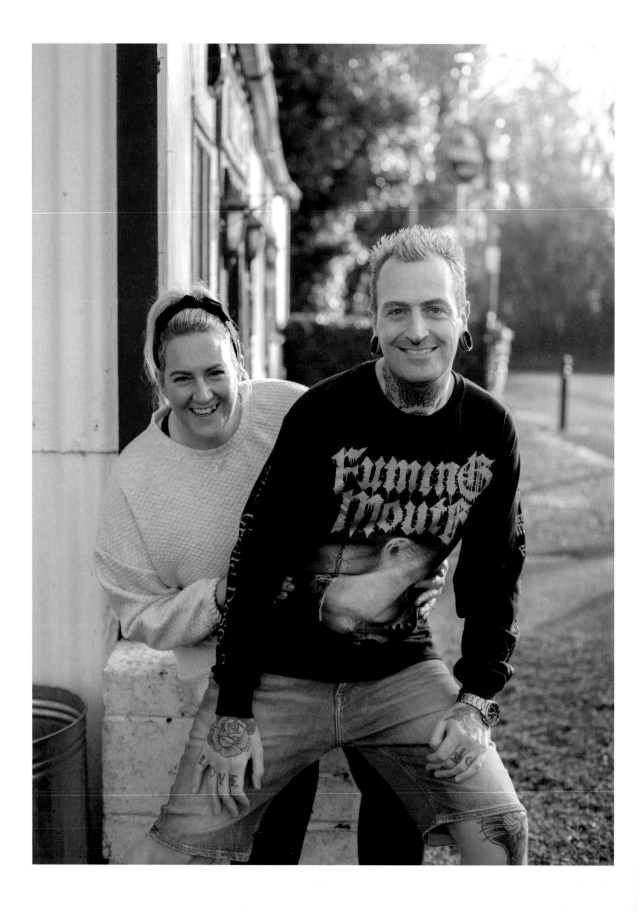

Leek and Potato SOUP

Another day, another hug in a bowl. There is nothing quite like a warm bowl of this old favourite served with some fresh bread and butter to dunk and devour. If you have some leftover chicken you can lash that in for some extra protein.

SERVES 4-6

Low-calorie spray oil

500g potatoes, peeled and diced

1 onion, diced

4-5 leeks, rinsed well and sliced into discs

1 litre chicken stock

100ml light cream

Salt and pepper, to taste

To garnish:

A small handful of chives, finely chopped

1 Get a large pot, spray with a little oil and place on a medium heat. Add in the potatoes, onion and leeks and stir well.
2 Fry off until the onion is translucent, then throw in a splash of water and let the steam soften the veg for a few minutes.
3 Add in the chicken stock and bring to the boil, then turn down to a simmer and cook for 10–15 minutes until the veg is soft enough to blend.
4 Remove from the heat and add the cream, then purée with a hand blender until smooth. Taste and season with salt and pepper as required.
5 Serve in warm bowls, garnished with chives, and have some fresh warm bread to hand for dunking!

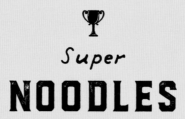

Super

NOODLES

Super Noodles were a firm favourite of mine back in the college days, along with a few cans of Dutch Gold. Well, fast-forward 20 years and here's a more filling and healthier take on them. This is basically a dish you can whip up using your store-cupboard essentials and transform a regular tin of soup into a masterpiece.

SERVES 2

1 small tin of sweetcorn, drained

Low-calorie spray oil

100g mushrooms, chopped

1 x 400g tin of chicken soup

200ml water

2 nests of rice noodles

2 tsp garlic granules

1 tsp curry powder

Salt and pepper to taste

1 Lash the corn into the airfryer at 180°C for around 10 minutes, or spread out on a baking sheet and put under the grill, turning occasionally so it doesn't burn, until charred and golden.

2 Give your mushrooms a spray of oil and cook in the airfryer at 180°C for around 15 minutes. Otherwise fry them off in a small pan until cooked.

3 While your mushrooms are cooking, put the chicken soup in a large pot then half fill the soup tin with water, and add that in too. Cook on a low to medium heat, stirring continuously.

4 Add in the charred corn and the rice noodles, being sure to get those noodles fully covered in the soup so they cook through. Add in the garlic granules, curry powder and cooked mushrooms and stir everything together. Season to taste.

5 Et voilà, homemade Super Noodles!

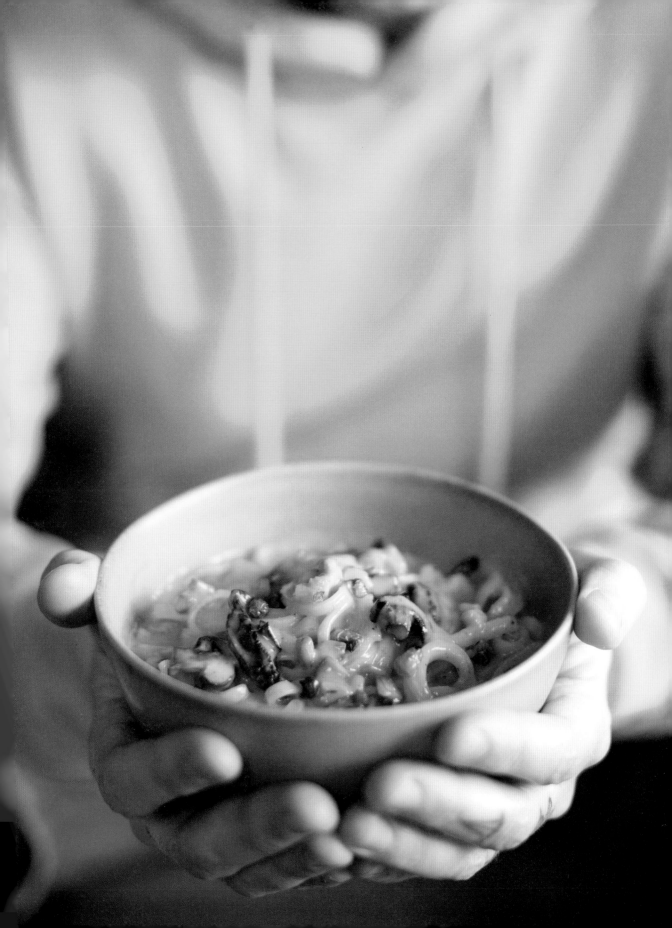

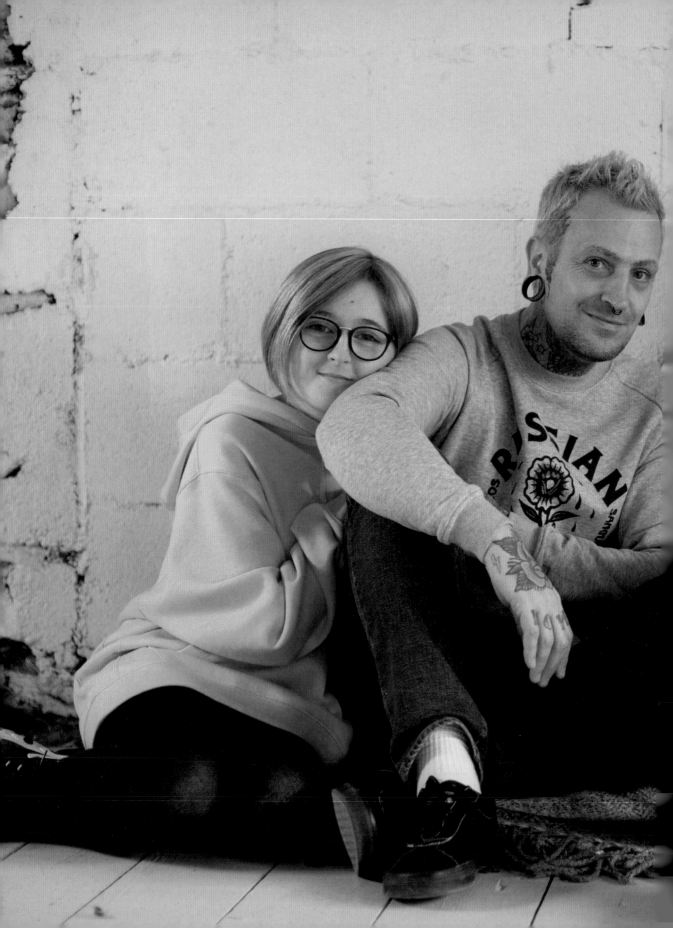

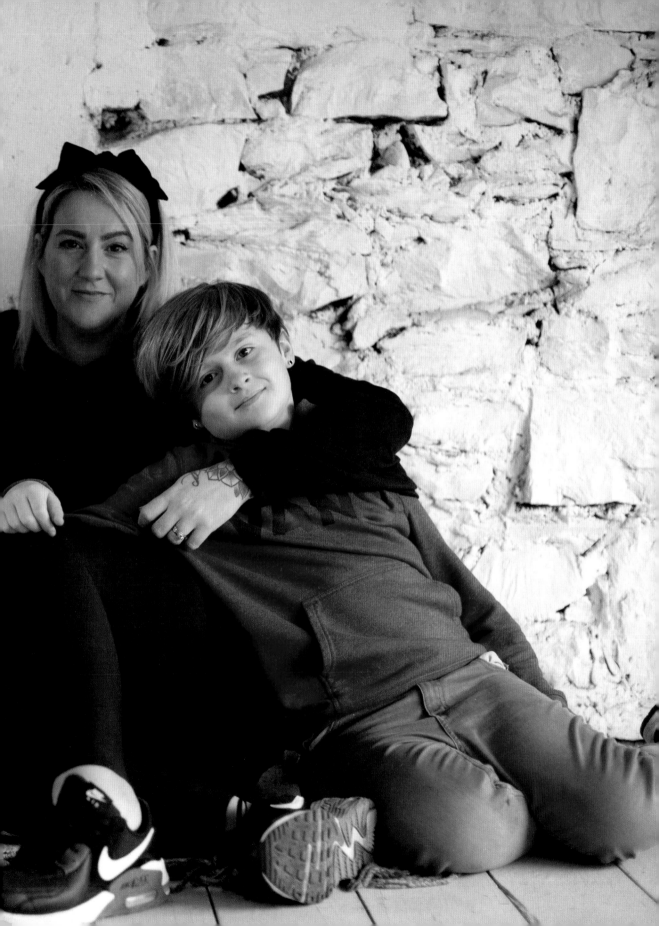

Ten-Minute Stew with Crispy
GNOCCHI AND EXTRA VEG

This warm and hearty stew is a ten-minute wonder. Using a tin of soup as the base will save you a ton of prep time but it will still taste feckin' deadly. I like to use as much fresh veg as I can but having jarred carrots and peas in the press can be a little saviour when you want something hearty but are short on time, stopping you from reaching for the crappy stuff!

SERVES 2

200g gnocchi

Low-calorie spray oil

1 x 400g tin of reduced-sugar chicken soup

1 jar of baby carrots, drained

3 tbsp petit pois, frozen or from a jar, drained

1 tsp mixed herbs

Salt and pepper to taste

1 If not using an airfryer, preheat the oven to 220°C.

2 Start by cooking the gnocchi in some boiling salted water for 2 minutes, then drain. We want to crisp it up now, so spread it out on a baking tray with a little spray of oil and pop in the preheated oven for 15 minutes. Alternatively you can pop in the airfryer at 190°C for 10 minutes with a spray of oil, shaking and turning halfway through until golden and crisp.

3 While the gnocchi are cooking, empty the tin of soup into a pot over a medium heat, then add in the carrots and peas, the mixed herbs and the salt and pepper to taste. Heat through for 10 minutes.

4 When ready, dish up in two warm bowls with the crispy gnocchi on top.

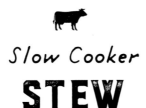

Slow Cooker
STEW

When I think of stew, I'm instantly transported back to my childhood, walking home in the pissing rain, wishing that Marie (my mam) would come to pick me up in the car, but she was probably too busy cooking up a storm to even realise it was raining. Then, getting to the front door and turning the key ... that was just left in the door, cause that's the way we rolled backed then (helllloooo robbers), walking into the hall and being met with the most incredible smell of comfort and warmth, it was literally like a huge hug. I wish my kids had got to taste and appreciate her stew, but they'll have their own memories of their mammy's stew. I hope they remember it like I remember my mammy's.

SERVES 4-6

Low-calorie spray oil

700g leaner option beef pieces

1 large white onion, diced

3 carrots, chopped into discs

1 kg baby potatoes, halved

2 tbsp plain flour

2 beef stock pots

1 red wine stock pot

1300ml boiling water

1 tbsp tomato purée

1 tbsp mixed herbs

½ tsp Worcestershire sauce

1 tsp garlic granules

½ tsp paprika

2 tbsp savoury gravy granules

1 Like most red meat dishes that I make in the slow cooker, I always start by browning the beef on a pan with a little oil. It's a step I try not to miss, as it removes excess fats and liquids, gives the meat a nice colour and adds to the flavour of the sauce in the cooking process.

2 Throw the onion, carrots and potatoes into the slow cooker and toss in the flour, mixing well to coat all the veg.

3 Then add in the browned beef, mix the 3 stock pots in a large jug with the boiling water, and pour that in too.

4 Pop in the tomato purée, mixed herbs, Worcestershire sauce, garlic granules and paprika and give it a good stir to mix everything together. Stick the slow cooker on high for 4 hours or low for 8 hours.

5 When it's ready I add my dirty little secret, 2 tablespoons of savoury gravy granules. I mix it in a cup with a drop of boiling water until it's a paste and then stir it in. This works wonders to thicken the stew and add an extra bit of oomph.

NICE
WITH
RICE

Easy Shredded
CHICKEN

Boiling chicken is something I have always done without a second thought as my mother always did it and my sister still does. But when I was showing it on my Instagram I got some mixed reactions about it! Although it doesn't sound that appealing, boiling chicken is a brilliant way to get tender, juicy chicken that will shred like a dream! Perfect for pulled chicken sambos or to add into curries or stews. Bookmark this page as I use this in lots of my recipes!

SERVES 2

2 chicken breasts

1 You can boil your chicken in water, seasoned with salt, or you can add a chicken stock cube to the water for some extra flavour. The choice is yours.

2 Put the liquid in a medium-sized pan on a medium heat (fill the pan about three-quarters full) and add the chicken breasts. Bring to a boil and simmer (keep the water bubbling) for 15 minutes.

3 Remove one fillet and check the inside is cooked through and not pink. Once ready remove both fillets from the pot and lay out on a chopping board.

4 Grab a couple of forks and shred them up. It's as simple as that!

Katsu

MUSHROOMS

A veggie take on the classic katsu curry! These mushrooms are absolutely delicious and can be either oven- or airfryer-cooked. If you don't fancy them with rice and curry sauce you can make them as a starter or a side dish with some yummy garlic mayo dip.

SERVES 4

1 punnet of mushrooms

50g panko breadcrumbs

2 tbsp lemon pepper

½ tsp ground ginger

1 tsp turmeric

1 tsp chilli flakes

1 tsp garlic powder

2 eggs

Low-calorie spray oil

360g long-grain rice

700ml curry sauce of your choice

1 chilli, deseeded and finely sliced

2 scallions, finely sliced

A pinch of sesame seeds

1 If not using an airfryer, preheat the oven to 220°C.

2 Grab two bowls so we can coat the mushrooms – one for the wet mix and one for the dry.

3 Put the panko breadcrumbs, lemon pepper, ginger, turmeric, chilli flakes and garlic powder into the first bowl, and give it a good aul mix.

4 Beat the eggs in the second bowl.

5 Dip the whole mushrooms first into the egg, then into the breadcrumbs, making sure they are completely coated. Repeat with all the mushrooms.

6 I like to cook the shrooms in the airfryer with a spray of oil for 20–25 minutes at 190°C, or you can cook them on a baking tray in the preheated oven for 25 minutes, turning halfway through.

7 While the mushrooms are cooking, cook your rice following the instructions on the packet, and warm up your curry sauce.

8 Once the mushrooms are golden and crisp, remove from the oven/airfryer. Serve them on a bed of rice, pour over the curry sauce and garnish with the chilli, scallions and a few sesame seeds.

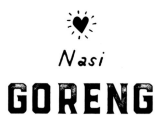

Nasi

GORENG

Nasi goreng is a delicious fried rice dish that originates from Indonesia. There are so many different variations but this is a super-quick and easy version and is ready in no time at all. I usually serve mine with a fried egg on top and with prawn crackers on the side to scoop it up.

SERVES 2

Low-calorie spray oil

2 garlic cloves, minced

1 bundle of asparagus, woody ends removed, and chopped into thirds

1 shallot, finely chopped

2 chicken breasts, chopped

3 tbsp soy sauce

1 tsp garlic granules

Salt and pepper to taste

320g cooked rice

2 tbsp mirin

To garnish:

2 fried eggs (see page 96 for my method)

1 scallion, sliced

Sesame seeds

1 Spray a frying pan or wok with some oil and heat. Add in the garlic, asparagus and shallot and fry off, then add the chicken, 1 tablespoon of soy sauce, garlic granules and salt and pepper and cook until the chicken is browned.

2 Next add in the cooked rice.

3 Mix the mirin with 2 tablespoons of soy sauce in a cup and add into the rice and chicken, stirring well until the rice is completely coated. Get your fried eggs cooking so they're ready for the garnish.

4 Pop half of the mix into a little bowl, and tip it out onto a plate, to give you a nice little 'sandcastle' of rice.

5 Top with a fried egg and sprinkle over the scallion slices and sesame seeds. Repeat with the remaining mix.

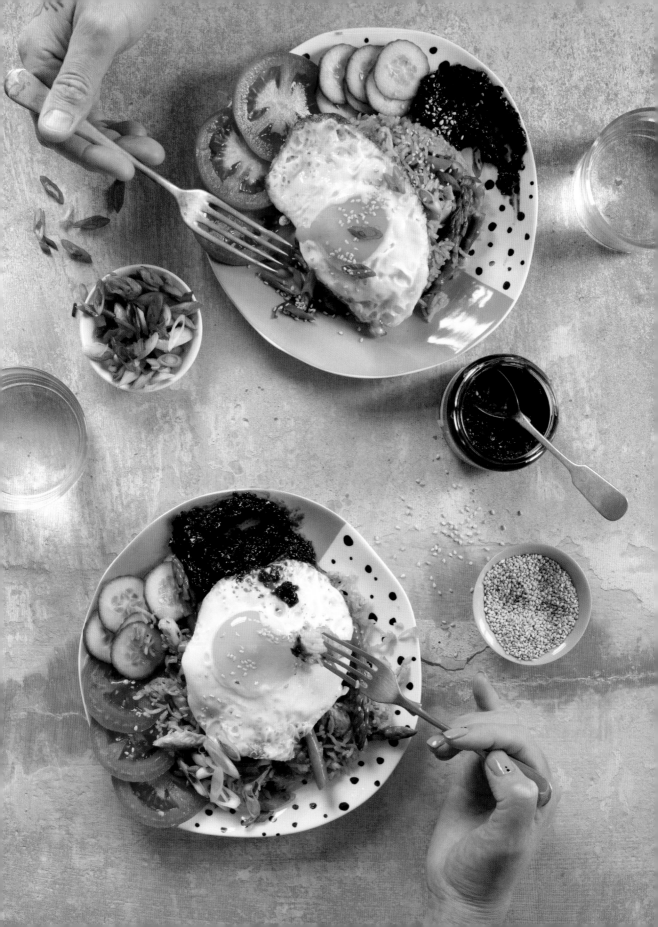

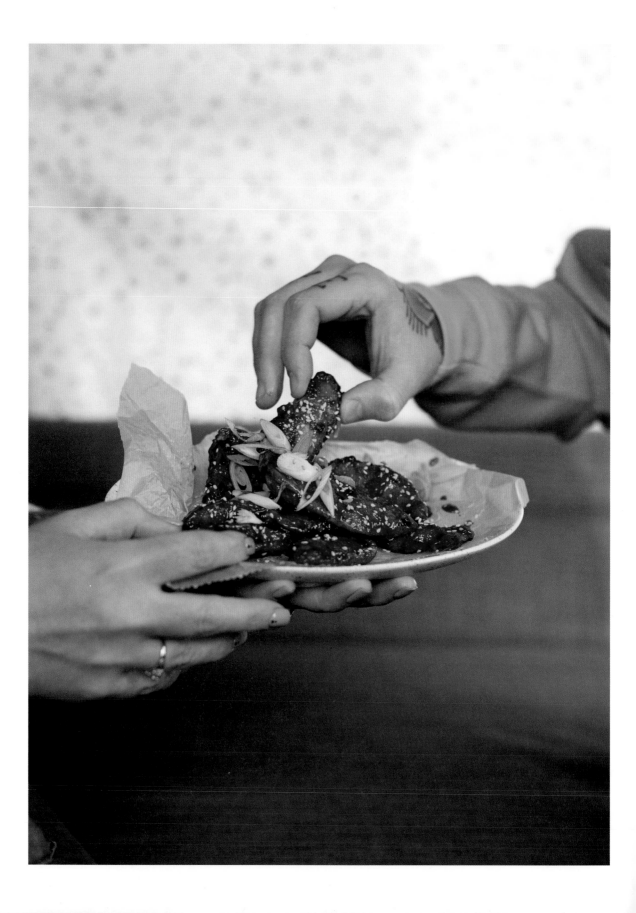

Crispy Shredded Sesame
CHICKEN

This has always been one of my go-to takeaway dishes and I'm so happy I can now make it myself at home. I always thought these dishes would be so complicated, but they are really easy to recreate and now you can enjoy a healthier version in the comfort of your home.

SERVES 4

3 chicken breasts, sliced into strips

2 tbsp cornflour

½ tsp chilli flakes

1 tsp ground ginger

Low-calorie spray oil

For the sauce:

3 garlic cloves, crushed

3 tbsp soy sauce

2 tbsp honey

1 tbsp sesame oil

2 tbsp reduced sugar ketchup

2 tbsp rice wine/white wine vinegar

1 tsp cornflour

To garnish:

2 scallions, finely sliced

½ tsp sesame seeds

1 If not using an airfryer, preheat the oven to 200°C.

2 In a bowl, toss your sliced chicken with the cornflour, chilli flakes and ginger.

3 Pop the chicken in the airfryer at 190°C for 15 minutes with a spray of oil until brown and crispy, or lay out on a baking tray with a spray of oil and cook in the preheated oven for 20 minutes.

4 While the chicken is cooking, get on with the sauce. Spray some oil into a wok over a medium heat, add the garlic, and fry off for 1 minute. Mix all the remaining ingredients for the sauce (except the cornflour) in a little bowl and pour into the wok. Stir and heat through until it starts to bubble gently and thicken; if it needs a little help to thicken up add in the cornflour mixed to a paste with a little water.

5 Add the crispy chicken into the sauce until nicely covered and glossy and continue to heat through for 2–3 minutes.

6 Sprinkle over the scallions and sesame seeds and serve with some boiled rice.

♣

Crispy Shredded Beef With

SWEET CHILLI SAUCE

Feck the takeaway and get your cook on with this deadly takeaway favourite. Gorgeous, crispy beef in a sweet chilli sauce and ready in no time at all.

SERVES 4

400g lean minute steaks, cut into strips

2 tbsp cornflour

½ tsp chilli flakes

1 tsp ground ginger

Low-calorie spray oil

For the sauce:

3 tbsp soy sauce

4 tbsp sweet chilli sauce

2 tbsp reduced-sugar ketchup

2 tbsp rice wine/white wine vinegar

2 tbsp water

To garnish:

½ tsp sesame seeds

1 If not using an airfryer, preheat the oven to 200°C.

2 In a bowl toss your sliced beef with the cornflour, chilli flakes and ginger.

3 Pop in the airfryer at 190°C for 15 minutes with a spray of oil until brown and crispy, or lay out on a baking tray with a spray of oil and cook in the preheated oven for 20 minutes.

4 Mix all the ingredients for the sauce in a little bowl and pour into a hot wok on a medium heat. Stir and heat through until it starts to bubble gently.

5 Add your crispy beef into the sauce and toss until covered, then continue to heat through for 2–3 minutes.

6 Pour out onto a serving dish, garnish with the sesame seeds and serve with some boiled rice.

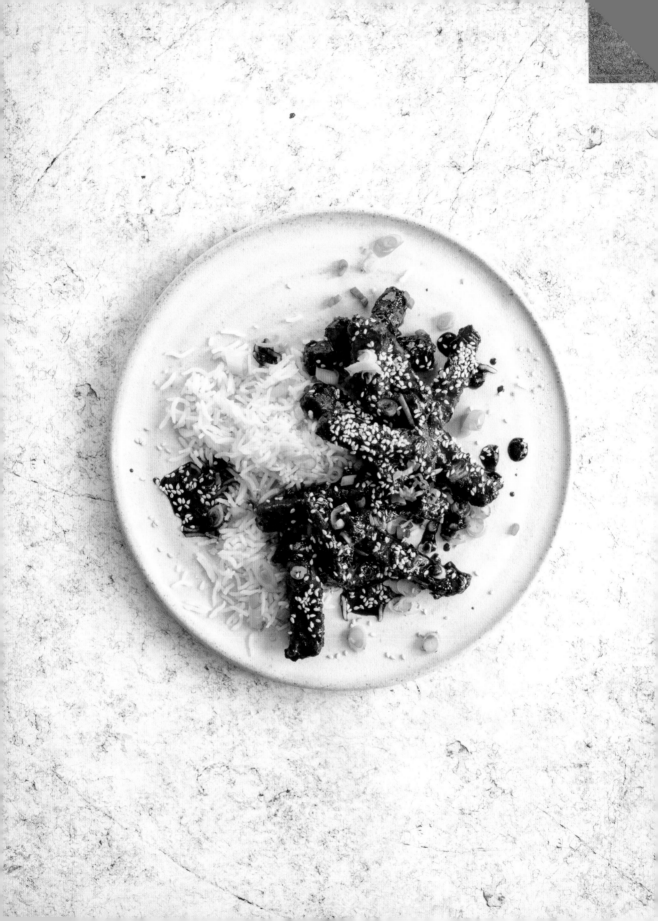

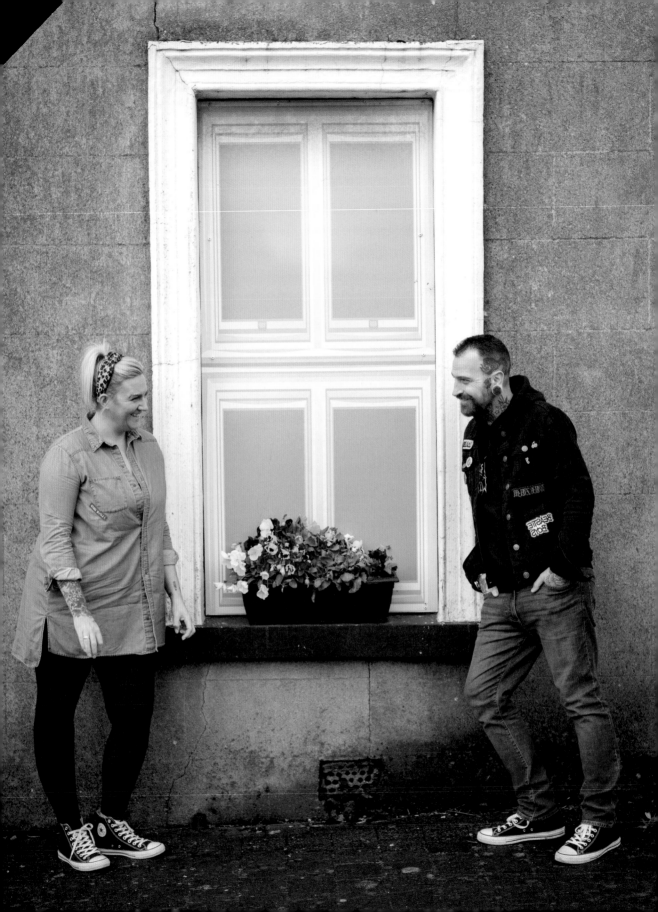

Crispy Chicken in
STICKY HONEY SAUCE

Another masso fake make that will quickly become one of your favourite dishes. This recipe has a mix of crispy chicken and crunchy vegetables tossed in a sweet sticky sauce with a whisper of chilli for a little bit of subtle heat.

SERVES 2

2 chicken breasts, chopped

2 tbsp cornflour

½ tsp salt

½ tsp white pepper

Low-calorie spray oil

1 green pepper, deseeded and sliced

1 small onion, chopped

For the sauce:

2 tbsp honey

2 tbsp soy sauce

1 tbsp sweet chilli sauce

1 tsp garlic granules

½ tsp ground ginger

¼ tsp chilli flakes (optional)

To garnish:

1 scallion, finely sliced

1 tsp sesame seeds

1 In a bowl, toss your chicken pieces with the cornflour, salt and white pepper.

2 Pop in the airfryer at 190°C for 15 minutes until golden and crisp, or fry in some spray oil.

3 While the chicken is cooking, heat a wok on a medium heat with a little oil and add the pepper and onion. Fry off for 2–3 minutes until the onion starts to soften but still has a bit of a bite.

4 Transfer the veg to a plate nearby and start the sauce. Put all the sauce ingredients into the hot wok, mix well, bring to the boil and simmer on low until it becomes sticky.

5 Add in the veg and crispy chicken and coat well in the sticky sauce.

6 Garnish with the scallion and sesame seeds and serve with some boiled rice.

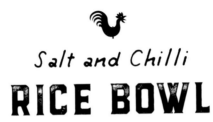

Salt and Chilli
RICE BOWL

This is kinda like a spice bag, but without the chips and meat – a nice veggie/vegan option that is ready in no time at all.

SERVES 2

Low-calorie spray oil

1 red pepper, deseeded and sliced

1 green pepper, deseeded and sliced

1 punnet of button mushrooms, sliced

1 fresh green or red chilli, deseeded and sliced

1 medium white onion, finely sliced

1 carrot, finely sliced

2 tbsp light soy sauce

½ tsp garlic granules

Sea salt to taste

250g cooked rice

Black or white sesame seeds

1 In a hot pan, heat a little oil and add the peppers, mushrooms, chilli, onion and carrot. Toss them in the pan and fry off for 2 minutes.

2 Add the soy sauce and cook for another minute, then add the garlic granules and a good grind of sea salt.

3 Next add in the rice and give it all a good mix in the pan, sprinkle with the sesame seeds and serve.

4 For an extra dimension, serve with a little drizzle of curry sauce! Absolutely mega!

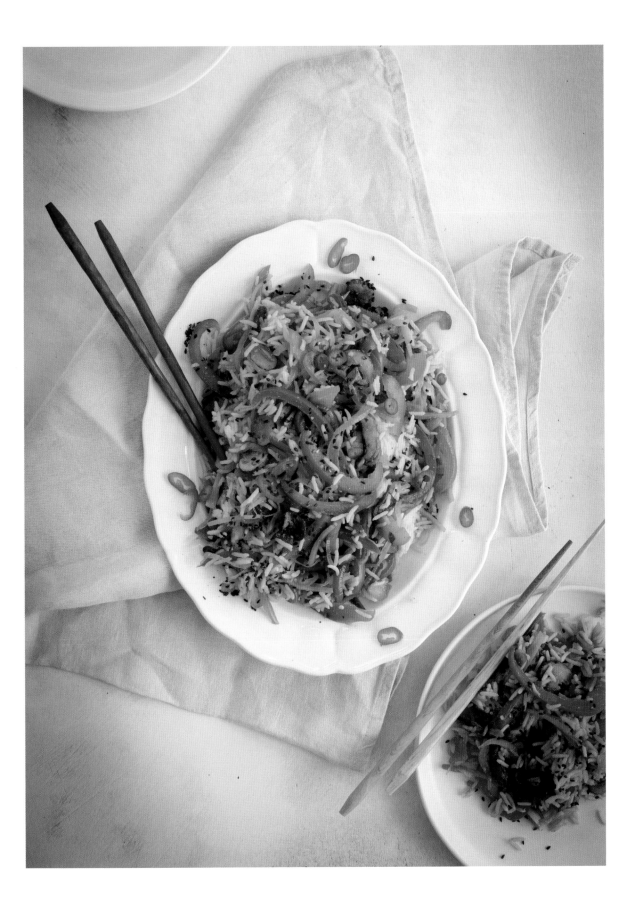

Sweet and Sticky

HARISSA CHICKEN

Simple, quick and bursting with flavour – that's how I like my dinners, and this recipe is just that. Using just a handful of ingredients, spiced up with some harissa spice, you'll be glad you didn't ring the takeaway!

SERVES 2

1 tbsp rapeseed oil

400g chicken breasts, chopped

1 onion, diced

1 red or green pepper, deseeded and diced

300ml chicken stock

1 tsp harissa spice powder

1 garlic clove, minced

2–3 tbsp soy sauce

2–3 tbsp honey

Salt and pepper to taste

1 tsp cornflour

To garnish:

Sesame seeds

1 Heat the oil on a pan, add the chicken and brown. Remove from the pan and leave to one side, then add in the onion and pepper, cook until the onion is translucent and remove to one side with the chicken.

2 Put the chicken stock, harissa, garlic, soy sauce and honey in the pan, sprinkling in some salt and pepper to taste.

3 Bring up the sauce to a boil then simmer until it starts to thicken. If it doesn't thicken add in the cornflour, mixed to a paste with a little water.

4 Add the chicken and veg back in and coat well with the sauce.

5 Garnish with sesame seeds and serve with some boiled rice or chips (page 6) – or both!

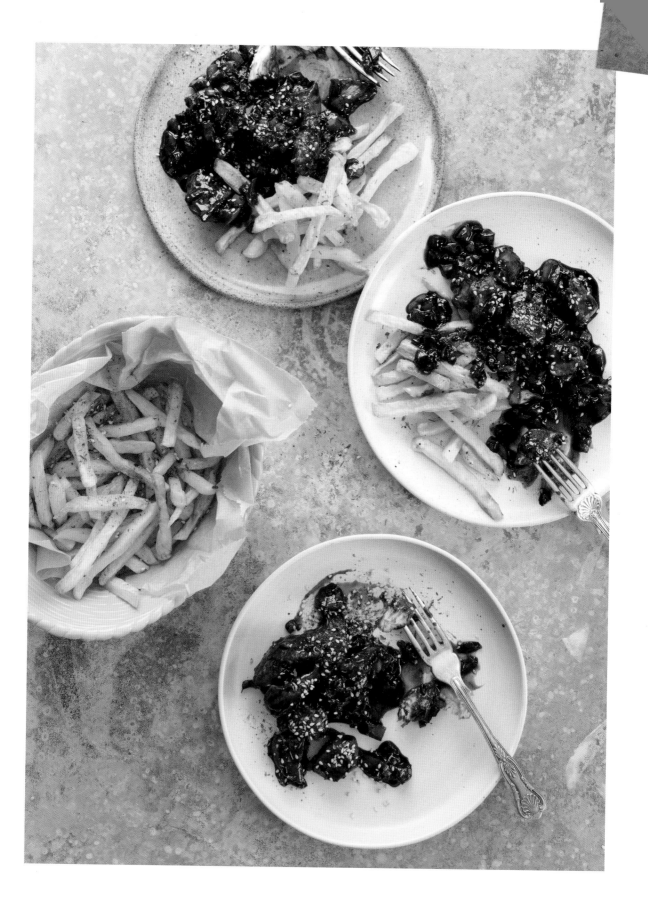

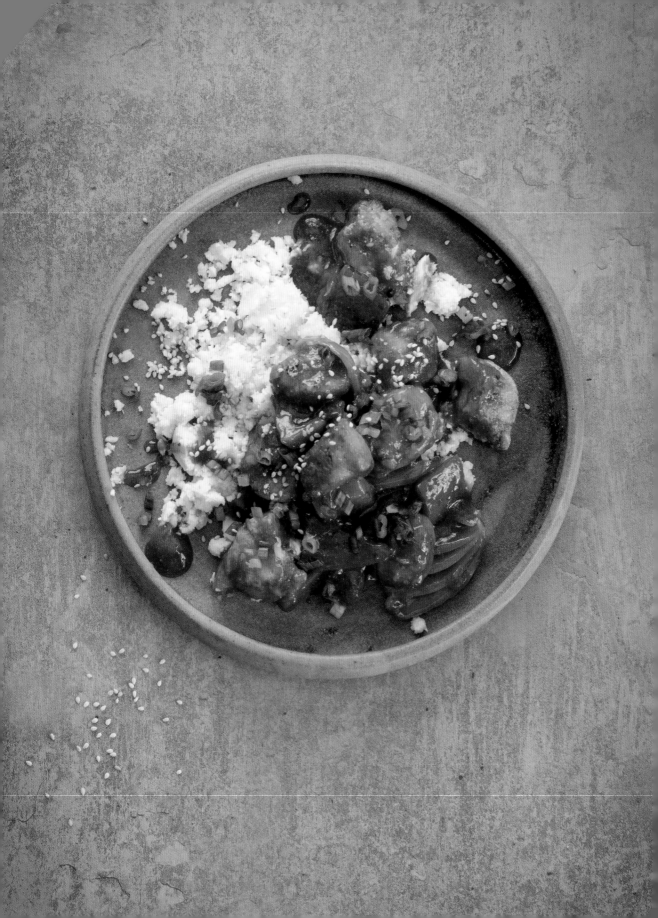

Zingy

LEMON CHICKEN

This recipe came about pretty much by accident. I had a bottle of lemon soy sauce sitting in the press just haunting me and I didn't know what to do with it until ... this dish was born! I've been making it on the regular ever since. It has a tang and is very zingy but that's why I love it.

SERVES 2

2 chicken breasts, chopped

2 tbsp cornflour

Salt and pepper to taste

Low-calorie spray oil

1 green pepper, deseeded and chopped

1 large white onion, chopped

For the sauce:

2 tbsp lemon soy sauce

1 tsp garlic granules

Juice of 2 lemons

1 tsp sweetener

½ tsp chilli flakes

1 tsp cornflour (optional)

To garnish:

1 scallion, finely sliced

1 tsp sesame seeds

1 Pop the chicken in a Ziploc bag and add the cornflour and salt and pepper. Give it a good shake until the chicken is fully coated.

2 Pop the chicken in the airfryer at 190°C for 15 minutes until golden and crisp, or fry in a pan with some spray oil.

3 While the chicken is cooking, heat a wok with a little oil and add the pepper and onion. Fry off for 2–3 minutes until the onion starts to soften but still has a bit of a crunch. Remove from the pan and start the sauce.

4 Put all the sauce ingredients (except the cornflour) into the hot wok, mix well, bring to the boil and simmer on low until it starts to thicken. If it doesn't thicken add in the cornflour, mixed to a paste with a little water.

5 Add the veg back in, along with the crispy chicken, and coat well in the zingy sauce.

6 Garnish with the scallion and sesame seeds and serve with some boiled rice.

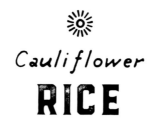

Cauliflower
RICE

This recipe is simply for reference – I wasn't clever enough to invent cauliflower rice, lol – but it's one thing I get asked about a lot on my Instagram so I'm putting it here so you can have a look whenever you need to. By the way, I absolutely love cauliflower and how versatile it is. Making this 'rice' is a deadly way to up your veggie intake with dishes that call for rice.

SERVES 3-4

1 head of fresh cauliflower, washed and dried and all green bits removed

1 You can use two methods to make the rice:
1. Literally grate it into a bowl just like cheese.
2. Lash it in a food processor and zap it until is broken up and fine like rice.

2 When you have made the rice, remove the excess moisture by pressing it in paper towels, which ensures it doesn't go all soggy when cooking.

3 There are two methods of cooking the rice:
1. Pan-fry or sauté with a little spray of oil for 5–6 minutes.
2. Microwave on high for 3 minutes in a microwave-safe dish.

4 The only thing about cauliflower is that it doesn't last well in the fridge – it will develop a funky smell. Best to make it and use it straight away or alternatively you can freeze it in a Ziploc bag ... handy!!

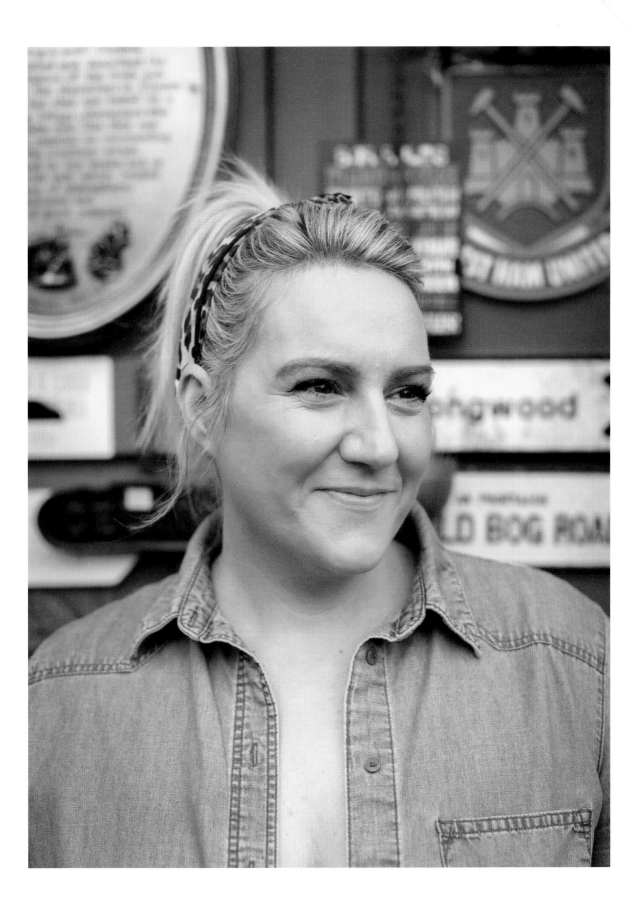

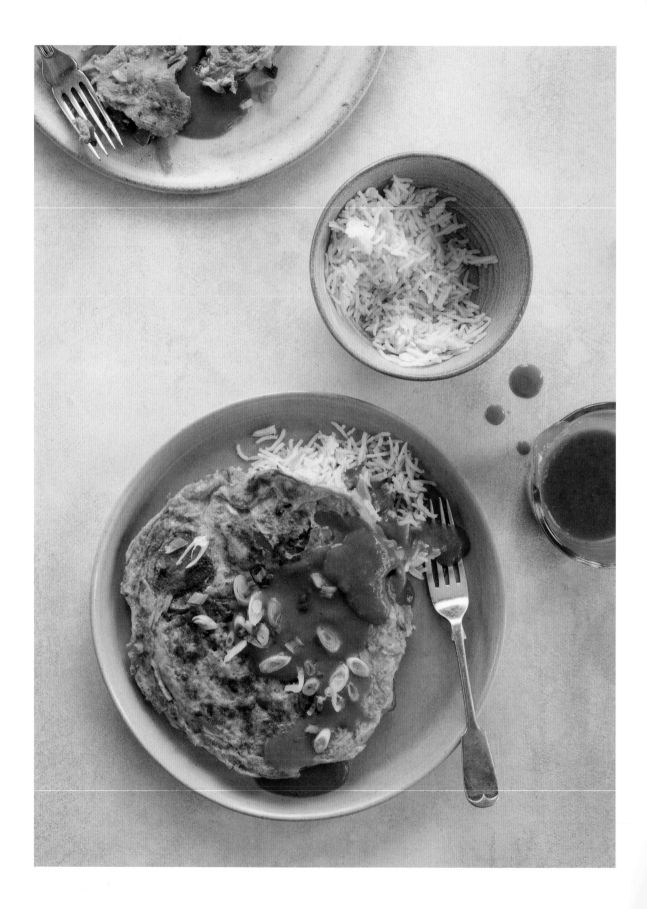

Egg Foo
YOUNG

For a brief period in my late teens I went vegetarian. Before this, my go-to in the Chinese takeout was a chicken curry so I needed to find an adequate and tasty replacement. The owner of the restaurant said I should try a vegetable foo young, which is basically a Chinese omelette. I got it with some rice and curry sauce and I was hooked. My vegetarianism lasted around a year or so and then I was back on the chicken curry like a good thing. I hadn't had foo young for years until I recently decided to recreate my fave dish from my veggie days. This recipe's a winner – quick and easy to make and really enjoyable. You can make it with any kind of meat too but I decided to stay true to my original veggie version.

SERVES 2

1 tbsp oil (I use rapeseed)

1 garlic clove, minced

8 mushrooms, sliced

2 scallions, sliced into small circles

1 onion, sliced

1 sweet red pepper, deseeded and sliced lengthways

100g beansprouts

6 large eggs

2 tbsp soy sauce

Salt and pepper to taste

280g rice (whichever type you prefer)

300ml curry sauce of your choice

1 Let's wok and roll – grab a wok, add a half tablespoon of oil and whack it on a medium heat, then add in the garlic and give a minute or so to fuse with the oil. Add all the rest of the veg and cook for a couple of minutes, mixing around as they cook to get them done evenly.

2 Remove the veg from the pan and put to one side. Get a large mixing bowl and crack in your eggs, add the soy sauce and beat together. Then add in the cooked veg and make sure everything is coated. Sprinkle in some salt and pepper to taste.

3 At this stage get your rice and curry sauce on the go so they're ready to serve when the omelette is ready.

4 Heat half a tablespoon of oil in your wok then add half your eggy, veggie mixture. Allow to cook for a couple of minutes then use a spatula or fish slice and turn. This doesn't have to look pretty and circular like an omelette – you just need to make sure it's cooked evenly. Repeat the process for the second one.

5 Serve the foo young on a bed of rice and drizzle the curry sauce over the top.

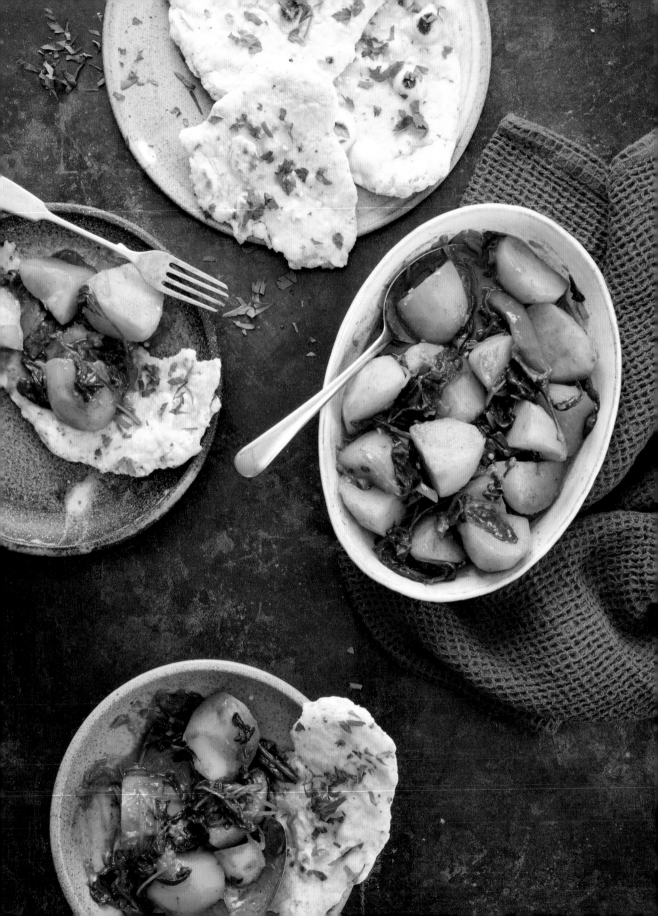

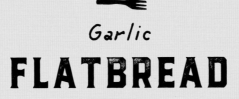

Garlic
FLATBREAD

Here's a simple, quick and easy little recipe that goes great with a curry or similar. Great to dip into a nice saucy dish. You can experiment with different herbs and spices but here we'll just keep it simple and use garlic.

MAKES 4-6 FLATBREADS

300g plain flour (plus extra for dusting)

1 tsp baking powder

2 tsp garlic powder

150ml water

Low-calorie spray oil

2 tsp dried parsley

Salt and pepper to taste

1 Grab a mixing bowl and lash in your flour, baking powder, garlic powder and water. Get your hands in and get mixing, until it's all squished together and doughy.

2 Dust your counter top with a little flour, break off around a sixth of the dough and roll it out into a small pizza-like shape. Continue with the rest of the dough, then give each flatbread a spray of oil and pop on a pan on medium heat for a couple of minutes per side. You want it to start going slightly golden.

3 Garnish with parsley and a little salt and pepper.

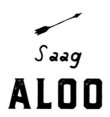

Saag
ALOO

Another favourite of mine from my old local Indian takeaway. I used to get this and some naan bread and dunk the naan in ... delicious. Well, here's a healthier take on it. Great as a side dish for a main or even just as a snack.

SERVES 4

500g potatoes, peeled and cut into small chunks

2 tbsp oil (I use rapeseed)

2 garlic cloves, finely sliced

1 onion, diced

2 red or green chillies, deseeded and sliced

1 tbsp ground cumin

1 tbsp turmeric

A 2cm piece of fresh ginger, finely chopped

½ tsp ground cinnamon

Salt and pepper to taste

250g fresh spinach, washed

100ml water

1 Pop your spuds into a microwave-safe bowl and give them a good wash. Whack them in the microwave for around 6–8 minutes; you just want to soften them up a little.

2 Grab a large pan, pop on a medium heat and add your oil, allow to heat up then throw in your garlic and give it a minute or so to infuse with the oil. Then add in your onion and chillis and cook off for about 4 minutes.

3 Next up, add in your prepped spuds, along with the cumin, turmeric, ginger, cinnamon, and a sprinkle of salt and pepper. Keep on a medium heat, mixing everything together for a few minutes. Throw in your spinach leaves and water, mix together and cover the pan. Leave on a low to medium heat for another 5–8 minutes, until the spinach is cooked. Delicious!

Prawn
TOAST

Another one of those fabulous starters or as I call them 'nibbly bits' that I loved to order from the takeaway. Typically, they are deep fried but my version is oven baked or cooked in the airfryer to give you a healthier twist but the same delicious flavour.

SERVES 6

6–8 slices wholemeal bread

250g raw prawns, shells removed

1 garlic clove, minced

A 2cm piece of fresh ginger, finely chopped

1 egg

1 scallion, finely chopped

½ tbsp light soy sauce

½ tsp sesame oil

100g sesame seeds

Low-calorie spray oil

1 If not using an airfryer, preheat the oven to 220°C.

2 Preheat your grill and toast the bread on one side, then set aside while you get on with the topping.

3 Put the prawns, garlic, ginger, egg, scallion, soy sauce and sesame oil into a blender and blitz into a paste.

4 Spread the prawn paste on the toasted side of the bread, sprinkle the top with sesame seeds and spray with a little oil.

5 Place the toast on a baking sheet and cook in the preheated oven for 15 minutes or until golden brown, or pop in the airfryer at 190°C for 10–12 minutes until golden and crisp.

6 Once cooked, slice the toasts into triangles and serve.

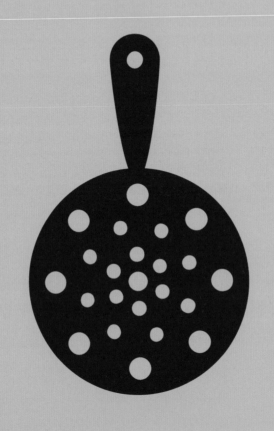

PASTA
BASTA

Chicken with White Wine and
HERB SAUCE

Here's a fancy one for you, perfect if you want to impress that special someone with a romantic dinner. So dim the lights, lash on your best Bee Gees record and get cooking.

SERVES 2

Low-calorie spray oil

350g chicken mini fillets

½ tsp smoked paprika

200g mushrooms, diced

2 leeks, well rinsed and finely sliced

400ml boiling water

1 herb stock pot

1 tsp garlic granules

150ml skimmed milk

100ml white wine

1 tsp cornflour

140g wild rice or dried pasta of choice

20g Parmesan cheese, grated

1 Fry off the chicken in a little spray oil then add in the paprika, mushrooms and leeks and cook until tender.

2 Measure your boiling water into a jug, then add your stock pot and stir to dissolve. Gradually stir this into the chicken, then lash in your garlic granules, milk and wine (100ml for the pot and 300ml for yourself, lol). Stir in and let cook for a couple of minutes.

3 Next up mix your cornflour to a paste with a drop of water and add in – this will thicken it up. Allow to simmer for a few minutes and it's ready.

4 Serve with rice or pasta, cooked according to the directions on the packet, and sprinkle over some freshly grated Parmesan. It's absolutely masso.

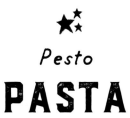

Pesto

PASTA

A simple but tasty pasta dish, this can be served fresh or popped into a container, refrigerated and eaten cold, which makes a great work lunch. It's so easy to make your own pesto – you'll never want shop-bought again – and you can fine-tune to your liking, adding in more or less of certain ingredients.

SERVES 4

A handful of pine nuts

Salt and pepper to taste

2 garlic cloves

40–60g Parmesan cheese, grated (plus extra for sprinkling)

2–3 tbsp squeezy basil (most shops sell this – it's dead handy)

2–3 tbsp olive oil

250g dried pappardelle pasta

8 cherry tomatoes, quartered

A handful of rocket leaves

1 Start by popping your pine nuts into a dry pan on a medium heat and lightly toast for a minute or so – you want them to get nice and brown, but not burnt. Watch closely – they can burn very quickly!

2 Transfer them to a blender along with the other ingredients (apart from the pasta, tomatoes and rocket). I always give my garlic cloves a quick crush with the side of the knife to make them easier to blend before I pop them in. Blitz until everything has come together and you have a nice, smooth consistency.

3 Next up, cook your pasta according to the packet instructions and fully drain, put into a pan over a low heat and stir in your pesto. Throw in your tomatoes and rocket, and mix everything together well, ensuring the pasta gets a good coating of pesto.

4 Serve with a light grating of Parmesan cheese and some salt and pepper.

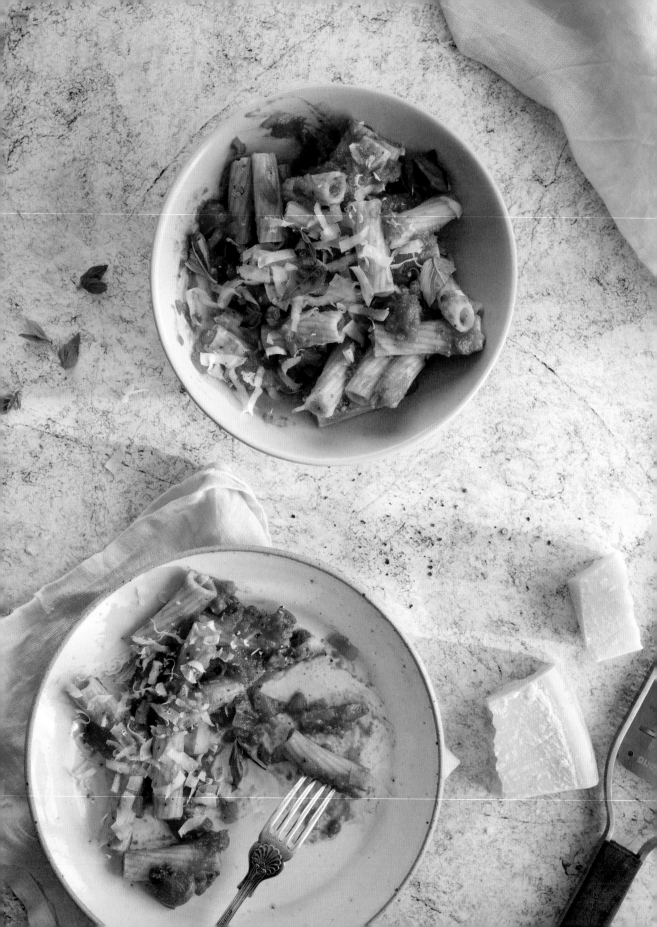

Arrabbiata

PASTA

This is a spicy little tomato-based minx, but if you don't like it hot, just hold back the chilli flakes and get it into ya! It's a handy one for the lunchbox for work too and can be kept for two to three days in the fridge. I used rigatoni pasta for mine but feel free to use any pasta of your choice.

SERVES 4

250g dried rigatoni pasta

5–6 sprays of low-calorie spray oil

1 onion, finely diced

2 garlic cloves, minced

1 x 400g tin of chopped tomatoes

1 tsp smoked paprika

1 tsp sweetener

1 tsp chilli flakes

½ tsp Italian seasoning or mixed herbs

Salt and pepper to taste

5 fresh basil leaves, torn

Parmesan cheese, grated

1 Boil some salted water in a large pot and add your pasta, follow the pack instructions for cooking time and cook until *al dente*. Drain in a colander and leave to one side until your sauce is ready.

2 While the pasta's cooking, heat your pan (I use a wok) and spray with the oil. Throw in your onion and garlic and sauté until translucent.

3 Mix in the chopped tomatoes, then add in the paprika, sweetener, chilli flakes and herbs and stir well. Bring to the boil, then reduce the heat and simmer for 10 minutes, seasoning with salt and pepper if you think it needs it.

4 Add in the cooked pasta and stir until coated with the sauce and heated through. Garnish with the basil leaves and sprinkle over some grated Parmesan if you fancy it.

Creamy
PRAWN LINGUINE

When it comes to fish, I'm not the best, but I do love a bit of cod and haddock and I absolutely adore prawns, so this dish always goes down a treat. You can used pre-cooked prawns but I like to use raw peeled ones, with the scaldy bit taken out – you know what I'm talking about!

SERVES 4

300g dried linguine
Low-calorie spray oil
2 shallots, finely diced
½ a 400g tin of finely chopped tomatoes
1 tsp garlic granules
200ml chicken stock
60g Parmesan cheese, grated
150ml light cream
300g raw peeled prawns
Dried parsley

1 Prepare the pasta according to the pack instructions, then drain in a colander and put to one side until your sauce is ready.
2 Get on with your sauce while the pasta's bubbling away. Spray a high-sided pan with a little oil, add the shallots and fry off until they are translucent. Add the tomatoes, garlic granules and chicken stock and cook for a further 5 minutes until the sauce begins to bubble, then turn down the heat.
3 Pop in the Parmesan and cream and stir through then add in the prawns and cook until they turn pink.
4 Add the pasta to the sauce, mixing until well coated and heated through. Serve immediately, garnished with some dried parsley.

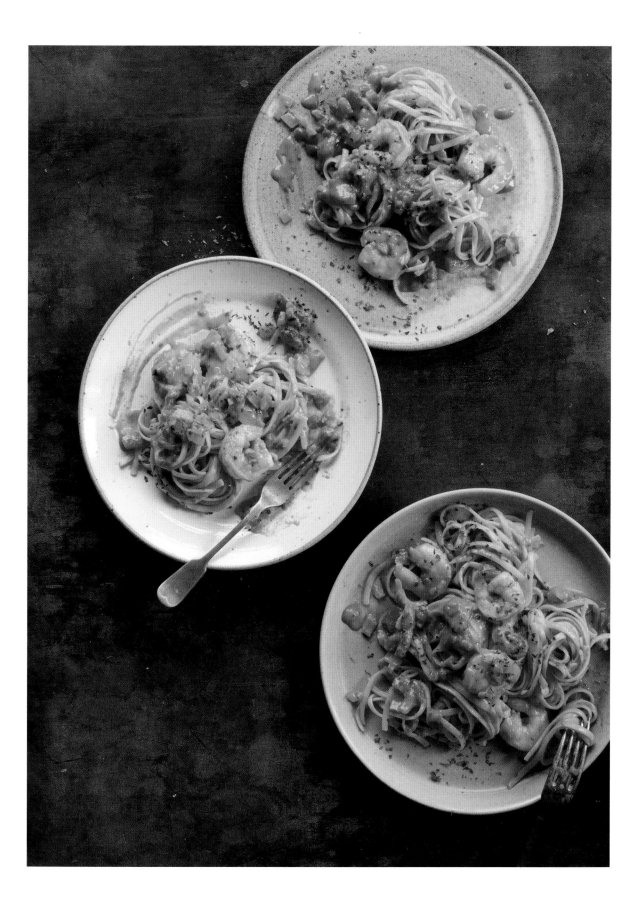

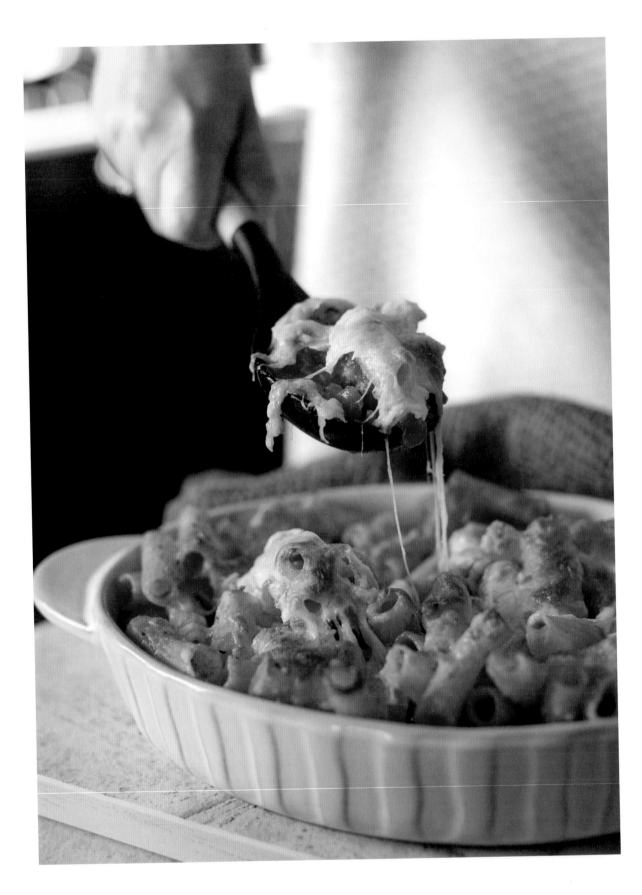

Tomato, Chorizo and Basil
PASTA BAKE

A comforting, rich tomato-based sauce loaded with pasta and cheese and a little kick from the chorizo – sure what's not to love? It's easy to prepare and can be made in advance if you have a busy day ahead. Super-handy to keep leftovers for lunch the next day.

SERVES 4-6

250g dried rigatoni

Low-calorie spray oil

1 onion, finely diced

3 garlic cloves, crushed

100g chorizo, chopped

2 x 400g tins of finely chopped tomatoes

1 tsp mixed herbs

1 tsp smoked paprika

1 tbsp sweetener

80g mozzarella, grated

30g Grana Padano cheese

A handful of fresh basil, torn

Salt and pepper to taste

1 Preheat the oven to 200°C.

2 Cook the rigatoni following pack instructions, then drain well, removing some pasta water with a ladle for the sauce before you do this.

3 While the pasta's cooking, spray some oil into a large pan and cook the onion and garlic on a low heat until the onion is translucent, then add in the chorizo and fry off for 2–3 minutes.

4 Add the tomatoes, mixed herbs, smoked paprika and sweetener and simmer for 15 minutes until it starts to reduce.

5 Throw in 50g of the mozzarella, all the Grana Padano, the cooked rigatoni and a half a ladle of the pasta water. Stir in well and simmer for a further 5 minutes.

6 Add in the fresh basil and season with salt and pepper.

7 Transfer the mix to an oven-proof dish, sprinkle the remaining mozzarella on top and pop in the preheated oven for 20 minutes until the cheese is golden and bubbling.

8 Serve and enjoy.

★ ★ ★

Vegetarian LASAGNE

This one is especially for my mother in law, Geraldine. She is mad for the veggie lasagne and she gave me her tips and tricks on how to create the perfect mix for this comforting, delicious dish.

SERVES 4

1 red pepper, deseeded and chopped

1 yellow pepper, deseeded and chopped

1 courgette, cut into chunks

1 sweet potato, peeled and cut into chunks

1 small punnet of mushrooms, sliced

1 large onion, cut into petals

1 bulb of garlic, top sliced off

Low-calorie spray oil

1 x 400g tin of chopped tomatoes

1 jar of garlic passata

1 tsp of paprika

1 tsp smoked paprika

1 tsp chilli flakes

1 vegetable or herb stock pot

1 red wine stock pot

1 tsp of soy sauce

1 tbsp sweetener (optional)

1 x 33g sachet of cheese sauce mix

Dried lasagne sheets

70g light mozzarella, grated

1 Preheat the oven to 220°C.

2 Lay out all your chopped veg and the garlic bulb on a baking tray or sheet lined with parchment, spray with a little oil and roast in the preheated oven for 20–25 minutes, turning halfway through, until browning and starting to caramelise.

3 While the veg are roasting, get a high-sided pan or pot and add the chopped tomatoes and half the jar of passata (you can add more if you like it saucy).

4 Add the paprika, smoked paprika and chilli flakes, give it a good stir then pop in the vegetable/herb stock pot and the red wine stock pot, letting them melt down into the sauce. Next throw in the soy sauce.

5 If you want to take the acidity out of the tomato base you can add the optional sweetener. Allow it all to simmer until the sauce starts to thicken.

6 Remove the veg from the oven and spoon them into the sauce. Get the garlic bulb and squeeze the soft garlic out of its papery skin and into the sauce too, taking care not to burn your fingers.

7 You can make your own white sauce but we love to save time and use a sachet of cheese sauce, made up with water in a small pot on a medium heat.

8 Now we are going to build the lasagne. Get a medium-sized baking dish and spoon in half the veg and sauce mix, cover with lasagne sheets and then add half of the cheese sauce. Repeat this process so you end up with two layers. Finish off with the grated mozzarella,

9 Pop into the preheated oven for 35–40 minutes or until golden brown.

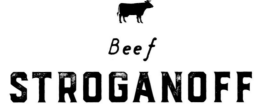

Beef
STROGANOFF

This is a recipe where you will lick your plate and wish you had seconds: an all-round family favourite that even the fussiest eater will love. I used to always buy pre-made sauces from the supermarket but when I started making my own, I never went back! Simple, quick and easy – just what you want!

SERVES 4

Low-calorie spray oil

1 onion, finely diced

1 small punnet of mushrooms, sliced

1 tbsp Dijon or wholegrain mustard

600ml beef stock

1 tsp garlic powder

White pepper to taste

2 lean beef medallions, sliced into strips

1 tbsp plain flour

2 tbsp light sour cream

250g dried pasta – I use pappardelle

1 Heat a pan and fry off the onion in a little spray oil until translucent, then add the mushrooms and cook through.

2 Add in the mustard and mix, then the beef stock, garlic powder and white pepper and bring to a boil. Turn down the heat and simmer for 10 minutes until the liquid starts to reduce.

3 Meanwhile, put the beef in a bowl with the flour mix until coated. Heat a clean pan with some oil and fry the beef until browned (I add some water to deglaze the pan towards the end so you get all the flavour from the bottom).

4 Add the browned beef to the sauce and stir in. Keep it on a simmer for another 5 minutes until the flour has thickened the sauce. Remove from the heat and stir in the sour cream.

5 While the sauce is simmering, cook the pasta as per packet instructions and drain in a colander. Spoon the pasta into the sauce and beef and coat well. Enjoy.

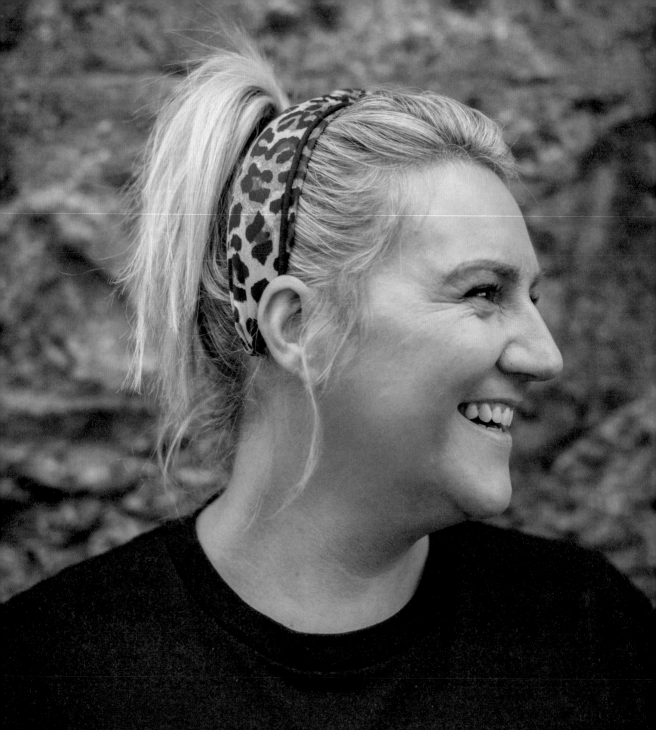

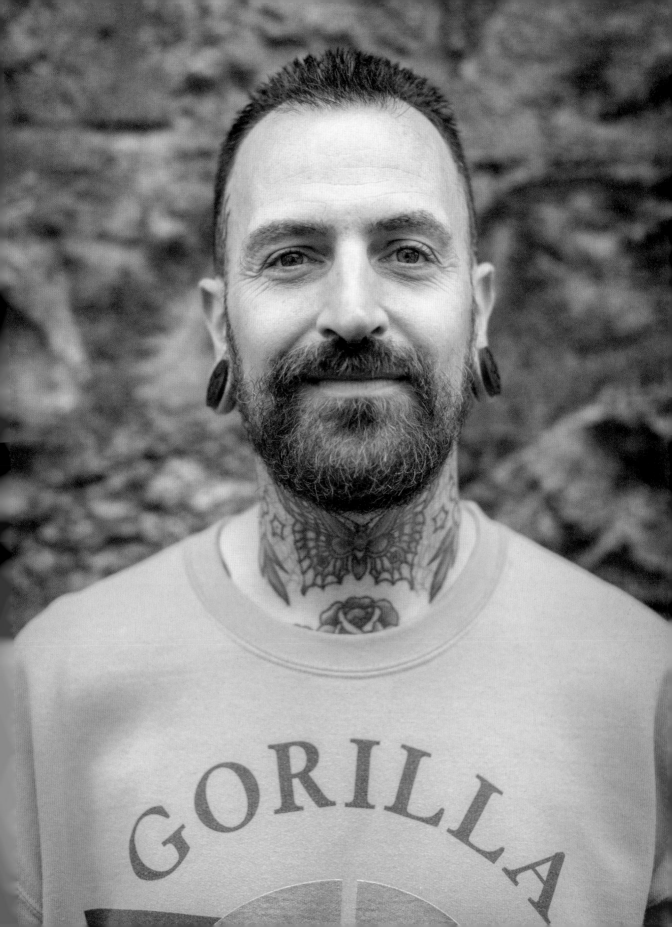

Slow-cooked
BEEF RAGU

Grab the slow cooker, lash it all in and all you have to do is wait! I make a 'soffritto' for the base of this. This is a typical medley of onion, celery and carrot used in a lot of Italian cooking. I make my own but you can buy a frozen version in some supermarkets.

SERVES 4

Low-calorie spray oil

1 onion, finely diced

2 sticks of celery, finely diced

1 carrot, finely diced

500g lean beef pieces

1 x 400g tin of chopped tomatoes

300ml passata

200ml cold water

1 tbsp garlic granules

1 tbsp Italian seasoning or mixed herbs

1 tsp sweetener

2 beef stock pots

A dash of Worcestershire sauce (optional)

380g dried pasta of your choice

1 I start by making a soffritto with the onion, celery and carrot. Spray a hot pan with some oil and add the veg – you want to cook them down until they become soft. I add 10–20ml of water every few minutes to help speed it up (traditionally a lot of oil would be used but we want to keep this a little healthier). Transfer the soffritto to your slow cooker.

2 I then brown the meat in a pan to seal in the juices and add this to the slow cooker too. Then just add all the rest of the ingredients (except the pasta), give it a good stir and cook for 4 hours on high, then a further 2 hours on low. If you are going to be out all day, you can just put it on low for 8 hours. When the cooking time is complete, the meat should be super tender and will break up or shred really easily.

3 When your ragu is ready, cook the pasta according to the packet instructions, drain and pop into the sauce and give it a good mix. You want the meat and the sauce to stick to the pasta so you get a bit of everything in each bite.

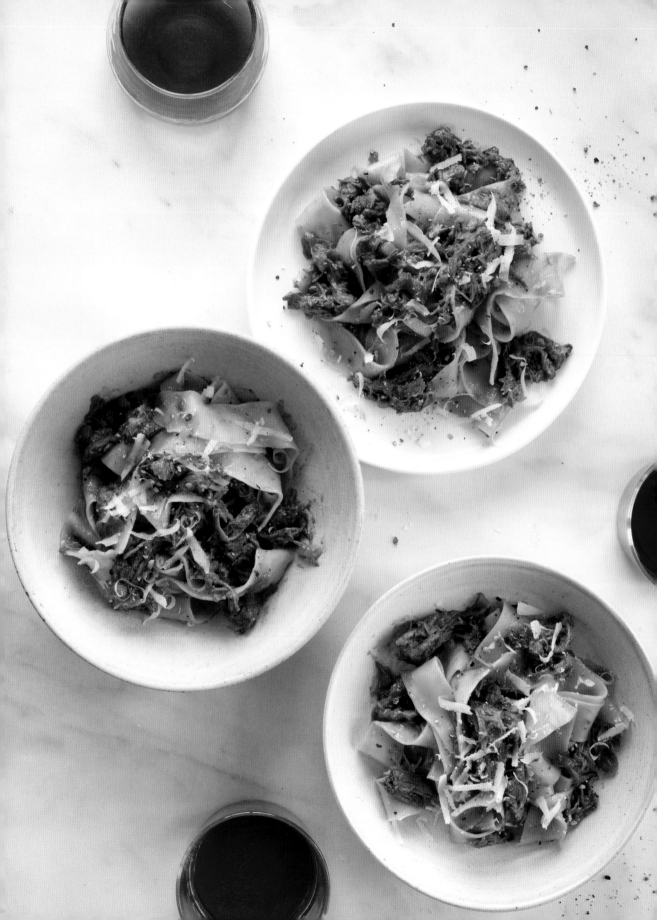

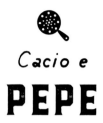

Cacio e

PEPE

I absolutely love Italian food; I love Italy full stop, and every time we've travelled there we've always had the most amazing food experiences. Here's a super-quick pasta dish that takes no time at all, it only has three main ingredients and hits all the right taste buds.

SERVES 2

200g dried spaghetti

Salt

2 tsp black peppercorns

60g Parmesan, finely grated, plus more to serve

1 Bring a big pot of water to the boil and season with salt, add your pasta and cook, giving it a stir every so often.

2 While the pasta is cooking, heat up a dry pan, add in your peppercorns and get them nice and toasty (but not burnt), you want to release all those awesome aromas – a minute should do the job. Throw them straight into your pestle and mortar and batter them to bejaysus (if you don't have a pestle and mortar you can crush them using a glass/cup).

3 Near the end of the cooking time, scoop out about 250ml of the pasta water into a jug, then drain your pasta when it's ready. Now you have to move quickly here (some banging tunes will definitely help you). Grab your cheese and 80 per cent of your crushed pepper, lash into a large pan and gradually stir in the pasta water (you shouldn't need it all). Keep stirring on a medium heat, you want a nice, smooth consistency, like white sauce.

4 When your consistency is right, add in your pasta and be sure to mix it all up with the sauce, getting it nice and coated. You can add in a little more of the pasta water if you need to. Add in some salt to taste too.

5 Lash your pasta into two bowls and garnish with the remaining black pepper and a sprinkle of Parmesan.

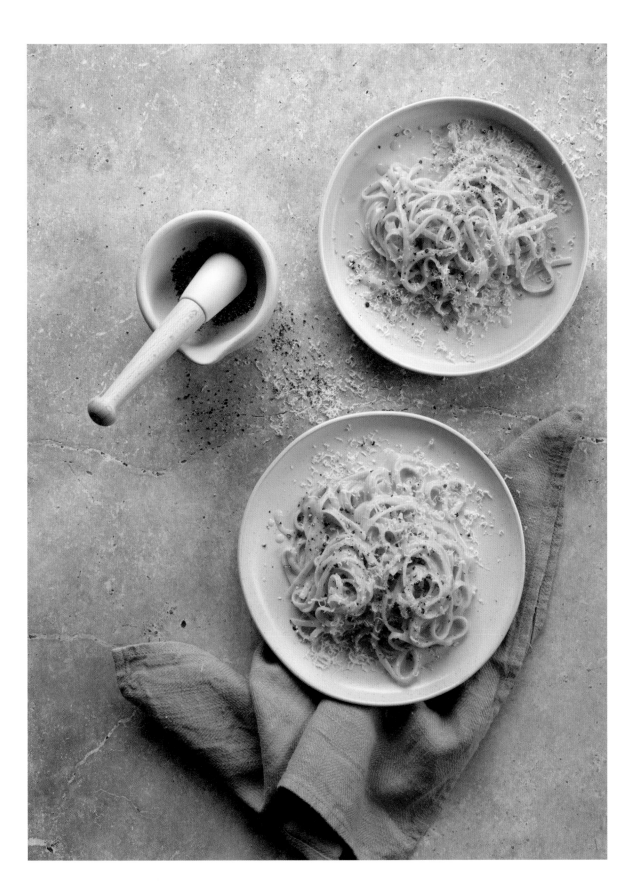

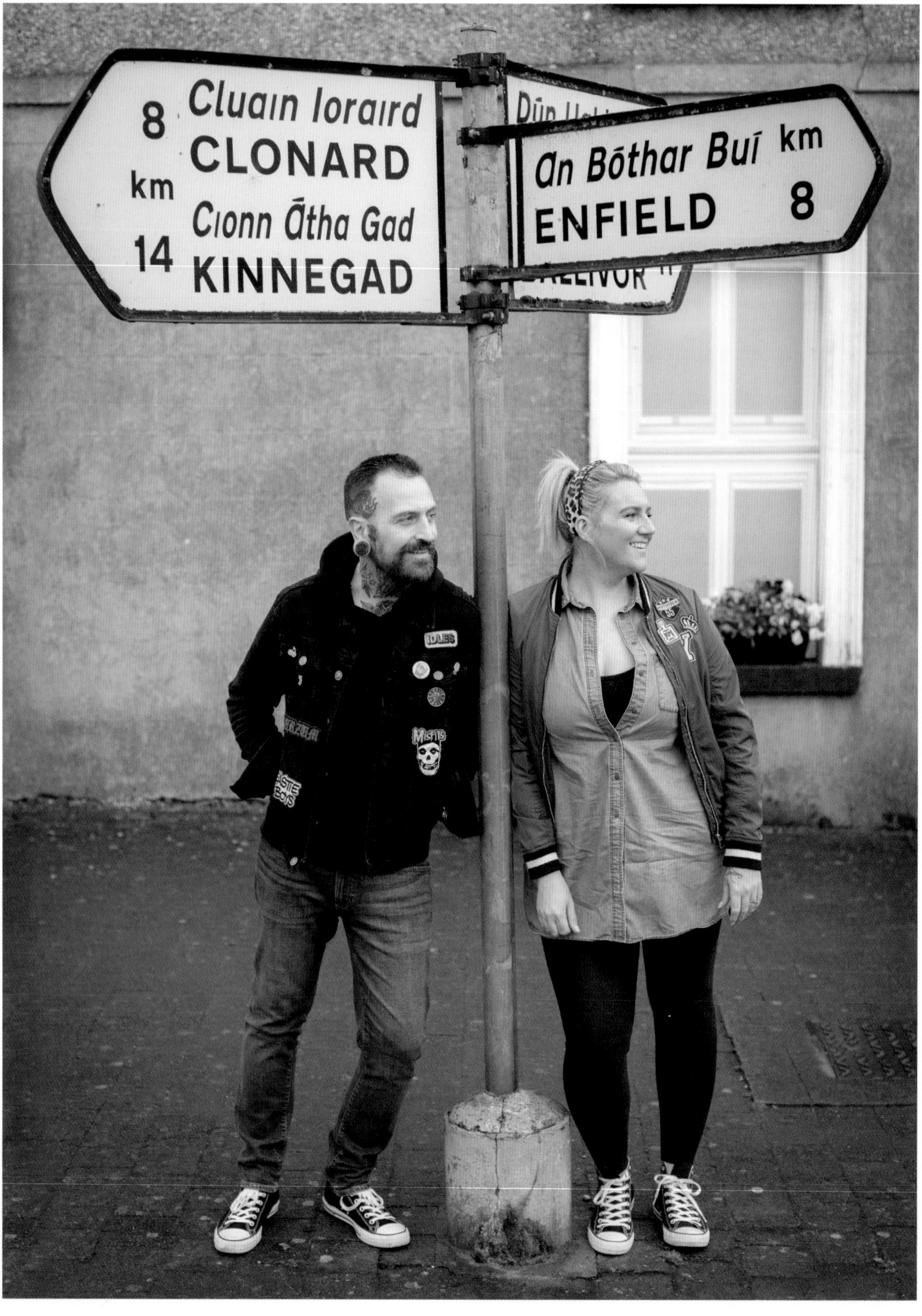
8
Cluain Ioraird
CLONARD
km
Cionn Átha Gad
14
KINNEGAD
An Bóthar Buí
km
ENFIELD
8
IDLES
MISFITS

ALFROGANOFF

This lovely recipe title is a mix of two of my favourite comfort dishes, alfredo and stroganoff. I keep this veggie-friendly but you can add meat for extra protein. It's tangy, it's zingy and it's just a deadly dinner to serve up. I like to use pappardelle with mine, but any kind of pasta will work just as well.

SERVES 4

175g dried pappardelle

1 white onion, finely diced

A large punnet of mushrooms, sliced

400ml beef stock

1 tsp garlic granules

50g Grana Padano cheese

1 tsp Dijon mustard

1 tsp cornflour

200ml light milk

Salt

1 tbsp light sour cream

1 Cook the pasta according to the packet instructions, then drain in a colander.

2 While the pasta is cooking, heat a high-sided pan and fry off the onion for 2–3 minutes, then add the mushrooms and cook, stirring well, until golden.

3 Pop in the beef stock and garlic granules and stir through, then lash in the Grana Padano and blend until melted in.

4 Next stir in the mustard, then mix the cornflour with the milk in a small jug and pour it in, stirring to mix.

5 Simmer until the sauce reduces and thickens, give it a little taste and season with salt if needed, then remove from the heat and stir in the sour cream.

6 When your pasta is ready, drain, add into the sauce and mix well to get every bit of pasta coated.

INDEX

NOTES

NOTES

NOTES

NOTES

NOTES

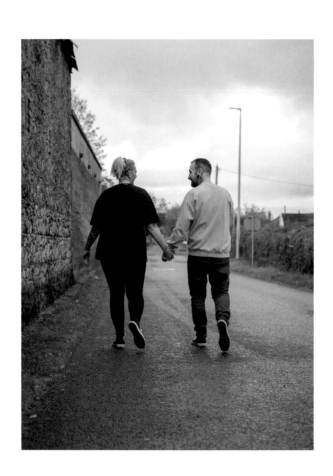